Güvenç Koçkaya – Albert Wertheimer

Pharmaceutical
Market Access
in Emerging Markets

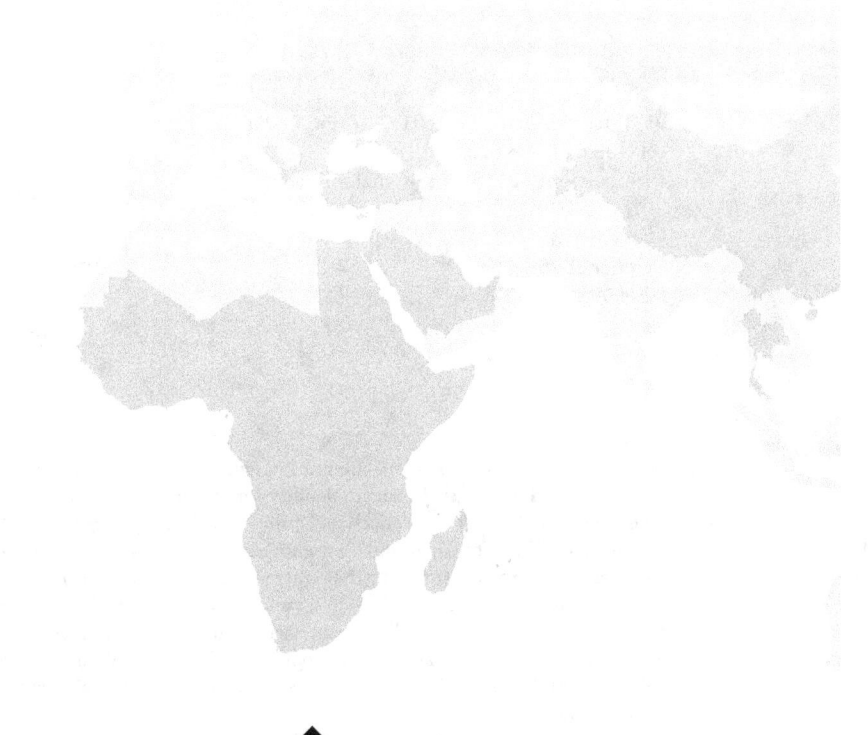

SEEd

Editors

Güvenç Koçkaya
Health Economics and Policy Association, Ankara, Turkey

Albert Wertheimer
College of Pharmacy, Nova Southeastern University, Ft. Lauderdale, FL, USA

© SEE*d* srl. All rights reserved
Via Vittorio Alfieri, 17 - 10121 Torino, Italia
Tel. +39.011.566.02.58
www.edizioniseed.it – info@edizioniseed.it

First edition
October 2016
ISBN 9781973307570

Summary

Preface 1

1. Introduction to the Market Access 3
Mondher Toumi, Szymon Jarosławski

  1.1 Origin of the Market Access term 3
     Market Access for goods 3
     Application of the Market Access concept to healthcare: similarities with market economy 3

  1.2 Healthcare market specifics 4

  1.3 Market Access definition..5

  1.4 Market Access key concepts 6
     What is Access...6
     What is Value 7
     Market Access and the structure of healthcare market...........................8

  1.5 Cultural specificities of Market Access 9

  1.6 Market Access from payers perspective 10
     The payers of healthcare...10
     Market Access tools to control drug expenditure 11
     The Value assessment by payers..12
     The link between HTA and Pricing & Reimbursement conditions..............14
     Non-HTA tools that affect pricing 14

  1.7 Market Access Agreements 15
     Definition 15
     Taxonomy..16
     The future 16

  1.8 References 17

  1.9 To know more 18

2. Market Access in Asian countries 21
Kally Wong

  2.1 Overview on the Healthcare Systems and Healthcare Policies 22
     South Korea...23
     China..24
     Thailand 26

  2.2 Recent Healthcare Policies 28
     Thailand 28

South Korea...29
China..29

2.3 Pathways of Market Access 31
South Korea...31
China..35
Thailand 41

2.4 Challenges and catalyzers for Market Access.......................................47

2.5 Market Outlook 50

2.6 References 52

2.7 To know more 53

3. Market Access in South American Countries 55

Arturo Schweiger, Alejandro Sonis

3.1 Introduction..55

3.2 General economic outlook...55

3.3 Health Sector 58

3.4 Pharmaceutical Markets..62

3.5 Health Technology Agencies 64
The History of HTA in Latin America..65
Red ETSA – Pan-American Health Organization (PAHO/WHO)...................67
How the future looks? 68

3.6 Market access..68
Mexico 69
Colombia...69
Access to Mexico...70
Access to Colombia...70

3.7 Final Comments 71

3.8 To know more 72

4. Market Access in South Eastern Europe Countries 77

Tarik Čatić

4.1 Introduction..77
Historical influence and heritage of healthcare sector 78

4.2 General Outlook of Healthcare System and Health Policies 78
Albania..78
Bosnia and Herzegovina 81
Kosovo 81
Macedonia, FYR..82
Montenegro...83
Serbia 83

4.3 Pathways of Market Access (Regulation and Reimbursement)..........84
  Albania...84
  Kosovo 86

4.4 Mapping and structure of Decision Makers...............................86
  Albania...86
  Bosnia and Herzegovina 87
  Macedonia, FYR..89
  Montenegro...90
  Serbia 90

4.5 Challenges and catalyzers for Market Access and Look-up for Near Future.....91
  Albania...91
  Bosnia and Herzegovina 91
  Kosovo 92
  Macedonia, FYR..92
  Montenegro...92
  Serbia 92

4.6 References...92

5. **Market Access in North Eastern Europe Countries**...................95
Esin Tuna

5.1 General Outlook of Healthcare System and Health Policies 95
  Russia...95
  Poland 97
  Ukraine 101

5.2 Pathways of Market Access 102
  Russia...102
  Poland 105
  Ukraine 107

5.3 Mapping and Structure of Decision Makers 110
  Russia...110
  Poland 111
  Ukraine 113

5.4 Challenges and Catalyzers for Market Access 114
  Russia...114
  Poland 115
  Ukraine 117

5.5 Good Examples from Successful Market Access Strategies...........118
  Russia...118
  Poland 119
  Ukraine 120

5.6 Look up for near future 120
  Russia...120

Poland 122
Ukraine 123
5.7   References 124

**6. Market Access in the United Arab Emirates and Selected Middle
     Eastern Countries** 129
     Ola Ghaleb Al Ahdab

6.1 The Middle East 129
     The Gulf Cooperation Council 129
6.2 Introduction.. 130
6.3 General Outlook of Healthcare System and Health Policies in the UAE and
     Other ME Countries 130
     The United Arab Emirates (UAE) 130
     The Executive Board of the Health Ministers for Arab GCC 133
     Kingdom of Saudi Arabia (KSA) 134
     Jordan.. 135
     Egypt... 135
     Lebanon... 136
6.4 Pathways of Market Access 136
     The United Arab Emirates (UAE) 139
     The Executive Board of the Health Ministers for Arab GCC 142
     Kingdom of Saudi Arabia (KSA) 144
     Jordan.. 145
     Egypt... 146
     Lebanon... 147
6.5 Mapping and Structure of Decision Makers 148
6.6 Challenges and Catalyzers for Market Access 149
     The United Arab Emirates (UAE) 149
     Challenges: Industry Perspectives 151
6.7 Examples from Market Access Strategies... 152
     Non Communicable Disease (NCD) – Patient Assistance Programs – Oncology,
     Differential Pricing Strategy 152
     Non Communicable Disease – Diabetes, Public Private Partnership Aimed at Capacity
     Building Through an Integrated Educational Platform 153
     Access to Innovation – 1st Oral Multiple Sclerosis Therapy Regulatory Fast Track
     Introduction.. 154
     Access to Unmet Need – Curative Hepatitis C Virus (HCV) Therapies..................... 155
     Non Communicable Disease – Diabetes, Payer Partnership – Disease Management
     Program 155
6.8 Look up for the Near Future 156
6.9 Executive Summary... 157
6.10 Acknowledgements... 158
6.11 References 158

7. **Market Access in Sub-Saharan Africa countries** 163
    Debra Leong, Mark Banfield, Anne Smart

    7.1 Regional Considerations for Sub-Saharan African Countries and South Africa
         as a Case Study 163

    7.2 Kenya 166

    7.3 Nigeria 167

    7.4 South Africa 167
         General Outlook of Healthcare System and Health Policies 169
         Pathways of Market Access (Regulation, Pricing, and Reimbursement) 172
         Mapping and Structure of Decision Makers 181
         Challenges and Catalyzers for Market Access 182

    7.5 Good Examples From Successful Market Access Strategies 184

    7.6 Outlook for the Near Future 185

    7.7 References 186

    7.8 To know more 188

8. **Market Access in Turkey** 193
    Fatma Betul Yenilmez

    8.1 General Overview of Healthcare System and Health Policies 193

    8.2 Pathways of Market Access (Regulation, Pricing, and Reimbursement) 194
         Pharmaceutical Licensing 194
         Pharmaceuticals Pricing 195
         Pharmaceutical Reimbursement 196

    8.3 Mapping and Structure of Decision-Makers 196

    8.4 Challenges and Catalysts for Market Access 197
         Challenges 197
         Catalysts 198

    8.5 Good Examples from Successful Market Access Strategies 198
         Good Manufacturing Practice (GMP) Audit 198
         Promoting Generics 199

    8.6 Look-up for Near Future 199

    8.7 References 200

9. **Comparing the Market Access and HTA process of Selected Countries
    from Different Regions** 201
    Mete Saylan, Özge Dokuyucu

    9.1 Introduction 201

    9.2 Comparing HTA systems 202
         Scope and perspective 202

Process and methodology... 203
Impact and outcome... 203
Quality... 203
9.3 Conclusions... 204
9.4 References.. 205

10. The Future of Market Access...**207**
Albert I. Wertheimer

10.1 The Market Access Avenues 207
Health Economics... 208
Knowledgeable Opinion Leaders (KOLs)... 208
Value Pricing 209
Value-added Services.. 209
Joint Education/Prevention and Screening.. 210
Personal Relationship Building 211
Softening the Gatekeeper 211
Advisory Boards.. 212
Other Market Access Endeavors 212
Pricing... 213
10.2 Conclusion 213
10.3 To know more 213

11. Conclusions...**215**
Güvenç Koçkaya

11.1 References.. 217

Glossary...**219**

Authors..**227**

Preface

The definition of Market Access was first reported by the World Trade Organization as "to open markets for trade and improve transparency, reciprocity and non-discrimination in international trade". But Market Access in pharmaceuticals is different than regular products like television, clothing, or cars. For these, the definition of market access for pharmaceuticals could be achieving the optimal price for a product or service and/or maximum reimbursement for the approved target population with no restrictions on funding for the medical technology.

By the way, market access is not only market authorization. It covers market authorization also, but more than market authorization including overlapping activities like pricing, health technology assessment, formulary and reimbursement. Especially pricing and reimbursement are the key factors of market access. Market access is one of most important activities for pharmaceutical companies nowadays.

Lets make examples;

- Think of a company that markets the most innovative products in the market. However, none of the products are secured through market access. Will anyone buy the shares? Possibly not.

- Think a patient where there is a current treatment available. However, her/his country`s MA process for the pharmaceutical is not finished yet. Can she/he reach the treatment? Possibly not and the suffering continues.

- Think a physician who wants to prescribe a pharmaceutical. However, the pharmaceutical is not covered under reimbursement. Can she/he prescribe it easily, especially an innovative high priced drug? Possibly not and again the treatment may not be available.

Depending on all these, market access is the key for pharmaceutical companies. We think these definitions are important and different enough to justify this book about market access. Emerging countries are important for the multinational pharmaceutical companies. It was reported that CAGR was 6.0 percent in the period from 2011-2017, and expected sales exceeding USD 1.1 trillion by 2017. In additional, CAGR 2008-2012 for recent launched pharmaceuticals were 9,8% for Emerging Countries and 1.5% for the top 8 developed countries. Depending on all of this knowledge, emerging countries can`t be ignored by multinational pharmaceutical companies for launching new products. So the market access process in emerging countries will be important in the near future also.

The market access processes in the most important countries in the selected regions are defined in this book and we hope it may help the local experts who are in the beginning or in middle of their careers, the government officers who are lookin for new implementations and examples from other countries, the headquarters managements who want to learn more about emerging markets.

Güvenç Koçkaya, Albert I. Wertheimer

Introduction to the Market Access

Mondher Toumi, Szymon Jarosławski

1 Origin of the Market Access term

Market Access for goods

The Market Access (MA) term was first introduced by the World Trade Organization (WTO) to define the competing relationship between the domestic and the imported products of a country [1].

The WTO defines MA as a set of conditions, tariff and non-tariff measures, agreed by WTO members for the entry of specific goods into their markets, that is to say the government policies regarding trade-barriers in general, and specifically the issues of import substitution (to promote local production) and free competition.

There are two types of trade barriers established by countries [1]:

- Tariff measures are taxes on imports of commodities into a country or region. Tariff commitments for goods are set out in each member's schedules of concessions on goods;
- Non-Tariff Barriers/Measures are any measure other than import duties (tariffs) used to restrict imports.

Whereas tariff barriers have steadily declined over the past few years, non-tariff barriers, such as technical regulations, safety or sanitary measures, have been increasing. Other non-tariff barriers are import prohibitions, requirement of a distribution network or effective means of marketing or of homologation for a product in a given country.

Application of the Market Access concept to healthcare: similarities with market economy

The concept of MA can easily be adopted for pharmaceuticals. For example, certification or homologation in the case of machinery is equivalent to the Marketing Authorization that is necessary in the pharmaceutical field in order to access a new market. Remaining trade barriers mentioned above also apply to the pharmaceutical market.

- Tariff Barriers on pharmaceuticals: As most countries import pharmaceutical products, they charge import tariffs, value-added tax (VAT), and other domestic taxes on these products to generate revenue and protect the local manufacturers from competition. E.g. Nigeria, Pakistan, India and China all have significant local pharmaceutical industries and are among countries with the highest import duties. The global trend has however been to reduce or eliminate tariffs and taxes on medicines in order to stimulate trade, competition, and the scaling down of prices [2].

- Non-Tariff Barriers on pharmaceuticals: Non-tariff measures have dramatically increased in the pharmaceutical field. The pharmaceutical industry is one of the most regulated. Complex measures range from marketing authorization, efficacy and safety controls, quality standards, pricing and reimbursement of pharmaceutical products, to import and distribution regulations, etc. Most governments have mandatory procedures to ensure the safety and efficacy of the medicines distributed on their market. Requirements for registration may involve specific local clinical studies that are not necessarily justified clinically. An increasing number of countries require clinical trials of a new product to be conducted or repeated on their territory. E.g. in China and Russia early clinical tests, as well as pivotal trials need to be repeated locally, which may take up to five years [3].

Finally, achieving positive reimbursement recommendation in countries with significant health insurance population coverage has become the most complex obstacle pharmaceutical companies need to face.

1.2 Healthcare market specifics

In spite of many similarities between healthcare products and other goods in a free market economy, the former is a unique field that challenges the traditional economic paradigm. There are four features that clearly differentiate the healthcare market from other markets.

- **The price is not determined by supply and demand**. In a traditional market economy context, the price is determined by supply and demand. A single entity assumes the functions of the buyer, the payer, and the consumer. In the healthcare market however, the prices are determined by payers through negotiation or are simply notified by the manufacturer. The buyer is the physician who prescribes the treatment, the payer is the health insurance provider, and the consumer is the patient. The three parties do not necessarily have convergent views on how healthcare should be delivered and what are the priorities.
- **Payers are committed to purchase health for the society**. The payer's intent is to provide health for the patient. When payers fund medicine they fund health production. They can only buy a proxy of health through the purchase of medicine and healthcare services. The actual outcome in terms of health improvement remains uncertain.
- **Health is specific to each individual**. Unlike food, real estate or technology, health cannot be shared or traded between individuals. The outcome of a treatment or a procedure also depends on individual characteristics of the patient [4]. The patients' characteristics may be not fully known *a priori* because of the lack of appropriate tools. This repertoire of scientific tools is evolving fast and changes regularly our understanding and approach to disease and therapies.
- **Externality of health**. Medicines can have a positive impact on the health of people, other than those who consume it. This is particularly the case for vaccinations

and antibiotics. The treatment and prevention of contagious diseases at the level of an individual can protect the global population from a potential epidemic: restricting access to healthcare for a subgroup of the population can have dramatic impact on that population health status; poor healthcare in a subgroup of the population will affect the health of the remaining part of the population that has good access to healthcare.

This is one of the main reasons for the creation of National Healthcare Systems. Illustratively, it has been iteratively reported that despite the highest per capita healthcare expenditure, the US do not have the best population health status, because of the wide disparity in access healthcare [5]. These disparities results largely from the lack of universal health insurance in the US. It remains to be seen if the Affordable Care Act of 2010 bring about desired improvements.

Market Access definition

The concept of MA in healthcare is heterogeneous and hard to define, depending on whether we are dealing with a private, public or a mixed healthcare system. It is the process by which a company gets a drug available on the market after obtaining a Marketing Authorization and by which the medicine becomes available / affordable for all patients for whom it is indicated as per its Marketing Authorization.

The following definition will be used in this chapter:

MA for pharmaceuticals defines the ability for a drug to achieve through a health insurance system a reimbursed price and a favourable recommendation for prescription.

It covers a group of activities intended to provide access to the appropriate medicine for the appropriate group of patients and at the appropriate price.

For the manufacturers, the ideal outcome of MA is to achieve the optimal price with maximum reimbursement rate for the approved target population with no limitation on prescription or funding procedures. However, in practice there is a trade-off between:

- Price and reimbursement conditions;
- Target population selection;
- Prescription and funding procedures.

Therefore, MA can be also seen as activities that support the management of potential barriers, such as non-optimal price and reimbursement level, the restriction of the scope of prescription for a drug or complicated prescription or funding procedures.

The scope of these activities is overlapping with the management of pricing and reimbursement, Health Technology Assessment (HTA) and formularies. The formularies are the lists of medicines that may be prescribed at the expense of the institutionalized payer.

Marketing Authorization from a regulatory agency, which could be the Food and Drugs Administration (FDA) in the US or the European Medicines Agency (EMA) in the EU, is issued based on consideration of the product's safety, efficacy and quality in the highly

---

Box 1. What Market access (MA) is not

- MA **is not** about obtaining regulatory approval (license, Marketing Authorization).
- MA **is not** about medical representatives getting access to doctors or pharmacists (sales force).
- Access to pharmacy shelves (distribution) **is not** MA.
- MA **is not** about choosing the right channel to promote product (e.g. marketing, Direct-to-customer advertising).

---

controlled conditions of Randomized Clinical Trials (RCT). In case of UE, national agencies are responsible for the implementation of this Authorization in its local settings [6]. Once a medicine is approved for marketing, HTA bodies are responsible for assessing its real-life efficacy (i.e. effectiveness), cost-effectiveness, relative efficacy, related medical need, budget impact and other evidence that will be later used by payers for pricing and reimbursement (P&R) decisions, as well as formulary listing and prescription guidelines.

Payers themselves are not qualified to evaluate those criteria, so they delegate these activities to independent groups of experts which produce the HTA evidence. HTA evaluations aim to inform payers' decisions and help them set the appropriate P&R conditions.

Finally, MA should not be confused with the activities summarized in the Box 1.

1.4 Market Access key concepts

If we consider the WTO definition [1], obtaining MA should be the ability to access the whole market in a given country, sell the product and achieve revenue on a market without obstacles. In case of pharmaceuticals, these obstacles are: Marketing Authorization; the P&R levels, logistics (storage and supply conditions), the drug surveillance (follow up on potential and actual product adverse effects) etc. In practice however, the pharmaceutical industry has become capable of addressing all those hurdles except P&R. Thus, for the industry MA has become synonymous to the hurdle of achieving high P&R levels.

What is Access

It is crucial to differentiate access from accessibility and MA. These are three different concepts, which are often misunderstood (Box 2).

Further, the stakeholders of the healthcare market have different objectives regarding access to medicine. While the objective of the industry is to provide the largest possible access to their drugs, the objective of the payer is to restrict access to the most beneficial patients alone, in order to achieve the highest effectiveness and cost efficiency. The industry must persuade the payer of the medical relevance and value of the drug to obtain access to a larger target population.

Box 2. Three concepts that differentiate access from accessibility and MA

- Access to healthcare or to health services is the perceptions and experiences of people as to their ease in reaching health services or health facilities in terms of location, time, and ease of approach. Lack of access: when a medicine is unavailable, inaccessible or unaffordable.
- Accessibility is the aspects of the structure of health services or health facilities that enhance the ability of people to reach a health care practitioner, in terms of location, time, and ease of approach.
- Market Access is the ability for a drug to achieve through a health insurance system a reimbursed price and a favorable recommendation for prescription.

What is Value

MA is related to the concept of Value for money from a payer's point of view. As a result, the primary objective of MA studies is to define and measure the value of health services and products.

In economics, value is a concept that refers to two different theories [7]. The first one is an objective theory, or the intrinsic theory of value, where the value of an object, good or service, corresponds to the cost of the production that is the cost of raw material and human work needed.

The other one is subjective and is more consistent with the idea of value as perceived in the healthcare market. This theory of value advocates the idea according to which the value of a good is neither determined by any inherent property of the good, nor by the amount of labour required to produce the good, but is determined by the importance an acting individual places on a good for the achievement of their desired outcome. The price offered is not a measure of subjective value; it is just a means of communication between the buyer and the seller.

As far as healthcare and MA are concerned, this last definition is the most relevant and should be used. In MA, the value of a drug or a health service depends on the subjective perception of the payer regarding the medical need in the society and how the product addresses that need.

This assessment of value made by payers is subjective, yet based on scientific evidence, such as clinical trials, epidemiology or cost-effectiveness studies. Most institutionalized payers formally require drug manufacturers and healthcare providers to submit evidence that corroborates the value of their product in terms of clinical outcomes and/or the cost of achieving such outcomes. Achieving a positive coverage decision and so, MA for a product, depends on the ability of the pharmaceutical industry to submit pertinent evidence. This calls for a thorough understanding of this evidence-based concept of value on the part of this industry.

The kind of evidence required by the payers for the assessment of a product differs from one country to another and covers a wide array of indicators, such as proof of clinical and economic value and more specific considerations of ethics, equity and/or politics. The focus of the payer is always on assessing the value for money of a product.

The set of evidence generated and presented by the manufacturer for the payer will form the value proposition. This term of value proposition is often used in healthcare economics. The development of such proposition is the ultimate aim of MA activities from an industrial perspective.

However, from a payer's perspective, the objective is to relate the drug's value to the right price considering all evidence. This is one of the most debated issues at the moment among various healthcare actors, and is often called value-based pricing (see sections "The Value assessment by payers" and "The link between HTA and Pricing & Reimbursement condition").

Market Access and the structure of healthcare market

Pharmaceutical markets can have a varying degree of fragmentation [8], from countries with a single national insurer to countries with multiple private insurers or a mix of both. In the latter two cases, securing MA is the ability to systematically gain access at optimal conditions in each and every area with each and every insurer. Depending on the type of healthcare market organization (e.g. centralised vs. decentralised or fully fragmented) the concept of MA may focus on different aspects.

Publicly-funded healthcare systems

Within publicly funded national health insurance found in most countries in Europe, the government defines the overall public health goals and corresponding funding usually through the parliament health budget vote [9]. Then, the rules for access to the market for the industry are laid out by a central agency or agencies. These involve the evidence requested for the assessment of a product and the criteria for making the funding decision. The public healthcare payers represent the society interest and try to integrate the society perspective when making decision.

Mixed or private healthcare systems

There are countries where the health insurance is fragmented and largely private, as in the case of the US. There is no unified framework to obtaining MA in the US and the public and each of the private insurers follow their own pathway. In this setting, private healthcare payers engage in independent negotiations with the industry. This can be seen a negotiation between two business entities that are looking to maximize their profits. However, in the US the public payers (the Centres for Medicare & Medicaid Services – CMS, e.g., Medicare, Medicaid, and the Children's Health Insurance Program – CHIP) represent an increasing proportion of the healthcare budget that is about to match to the commercial. The CMS pathway resembles that of many European countries, Australia or Canada, except that formal health-economic analysis or HTA are not compulsory in the US, except very rare cases. Further, high cost should not be a cause for a negative reimbursement advice by the CMS.

Centralized and regional Market Access

A trend towards decentralization is emerging also in the public healthcare settings, as policy-making is increasingly devolved from the national bodies to local health authorities [10]. As healthcare payers are compelled to curb their pharmaceutical budgets, in a context of economic crisis, local policy makers are also exacted to decide on which therapies are funded, and under what conditions. However, these responsibilities are not always matched with competences at the regional level. In many countries, the regional authorities accountable for medicine spending are seldom prepared to negotiate the costs of the drugs or to assess their value. Concomitantly, there is increasing incitement to concentrate on cost-containment of the healthcare budgets they hold.

This trend is blurring the traditional division between countries with decentralized healthcare systems, such as Spain, Italy, Sweden or Germany and countries with more centralized ones, like France or England. E.g. in England, where strategic decisions affecting the National Health System remain in the authority of the National Department of Health, the power of execution is assigned to a large number of Primary Care Trusts (PCTs). Each PCT is responsible for the provision and funding of healthcare services for populations that range from 90,000 to over 1,259,000 individuals. Concretely, this means that, apart from the national bodies, the pharmaceutical industry has to engage directly with PCTs, in order to access the markets in England.

Cultural specificities of Market Access

The MA strategy needs to be culturally-sensitive, even among countries that seemingly apply the same methodology to inform their drug funding decisions. E.g. countries in

	France [11]	Germany [12]	UK [13]
Objective	Secure access to all new products, but at the right price	Obtain savings on drug spending with no detriment to safety/efficacy	Obtain rational allocation of resources
Process	Driver: Public health relevance of benefit compared to the next best alternative Method: Single double blind randomized clinical trial Effect size	Driver: Same effect - same price (e.g. jumbo groups) Method: Meta-analysis Efficiency frontier as a back up	Driver: Maximization of efficiency of the health care output Method: Cost utility Threshold is 30,000 £/QALY
Impact	Gate-keeper for market entry	Reimbursement level	Recommendation for prescriber Formulary listing

Table 1. Cultural differences between authorities in EU countries regarding the objective, the process and the impact of HTA evaluation in MA
QALY: Quality-Adjusted Life Year

Northern Europe (UK, Scandinavia, The Netherlands)
- **Prescribers** follow gudilines and recommendations form National Health Insurance and are willing to accept cost containment measures
- **Payers** use cost-effectivness to support decissions and prefer restriction of drug recommendation to subpopulations of patients

Southern Europe (France, Italy, Spain)
- **Prescribers** behaviour is difficult to control by National Health Insurance
- **Payers** use efficacy to support decissions and prefer to negotiate lower price with manufacturer rather than restrict drug use to subpopulations of patients

Figure 1. The cultural differences among prescribers and payers in Europe

Europe that employ formal HTA can still substantially differ in the objective, the process and the impact of the HTA in MA (Table 1).

Finally, in Europe there is a geographical dichotomy between the northern and southern European countries, the former being more centralised and reluctant to price negotiation (Figure 1).

1.6 Market Access from payers perspective

The payers of healthcare

In healthcare, payers are generally entities that finance or reimburse the cost of health services. In the healthcare market, payers always act as gatekeepers for MA.

In most European countries, there is one main payer in each country, corresponding to the national public health insurance. Sometimes, there are additional payers at a regional level, or a mix of national and fragmented private payers as in the US. Importantly, each payer can have different objectives, perspectives and processes.

Depending on the country and level of authority, payers can be [10]:
- Members of national pricing committees (for example, France, Italy, Spain) and other key staff of the national health insurer;
- Members of HTA committees, either national (UK, Germany) or regional HTA bodies (Spain, Sweden);
- General practitioners in the UK and Germany, where doctors are paid by performance – their remuneration is linked to cost-containing prescription behaviour;
- Private health insurers (analogous to national insurers, but under smaller political pressure);
- Pharmacists in some countries (particularly chief pharmacists in the UK);
- Hospital managers and hospital staff with whom payers interact;

- Employers who pay for health insurance plans.
- Payers should not be considered as a homogeneous audience, but rather as a complex and heterogeneous one. The arguments accepted by one payer may be counterproductive for another payer within the same country.

Market Access tools to control drug expenditure

The continuous growth of healthcare expenditure and more specifically pharmaceutical expenditure has put healthcare insurance providers under escalating pressure. For payers, MA tools are a powerful way to control drug expenditures [14].

Despite an increasing proportion of products for which cheaper generic versions exist, the pharmaceutical market value continues to grow. To tackle this growth, payers have employed a variety of cost containment measures since the late '90. Nevertheless, they failed to control the growth of expenditure. In OECD (Organisation for Economic Co-operation and Development) countries, excluding the US, healthcare spending has almost doubled its share of GDP (Gross Domestic Product) over the last 10 years. The demographic changes and the expected future innovations are expected to generate a disruptive pressure unless appropriate action is taken. Pharmaceutical growth is a lot more significant than the healthcare growth, and accounts for as high as 20% in many developed countries.

The most common regulation of drug expenditure is price control. The institutionalized payer decides on the appropriate price of a medicine after negotiation with the marketing authorization holder. Only two countries still enjoy the free (uncontrolled) pricing process: USA, and UK. However, the two countries have put in place a number of regulatory processes that indirectly regulate prices. I.e. if a drug is thought to be overpriced, the access to the market is narrowed by means of negative list recommendations (UK). Free pricing in the UK was supposed to be replaced by a controlled pricing process, following the recommendation of the UK's Office of Fair Trading (OFT). Although the initiative of value based pricing failed, the new way to control pharmaceutical product prices have become for pharmaceutical companies to offer very high discounts that remain confidential but are often above 50% of listed price.

Other pharmaceutical cost-containment measures developed by payers include general price cuts, reference pricing (see section "Non-HTA tools that affect pricing") or exceptional taxes on turnover and profit.

During the 90s, the pricing regulation in Europe was often based on the health authorities' subjective perception of what the right price was. In order to dissolve political pressure around patients' access to new medicines and incentives for the industry to innovate, the authorities needed to implement more clear and objective rules for establishing prices. This resulted in two key developments:

- The creation of national HTA bodies across EU countries, Australia and Canada that assess evidence supporting the benefit of new medicines and other health technologies;
- The creation of reference pricing within therapeutic class and across EU countries (see section "Non-HTA tools that affect pricing").

- This trend is also seen in the US where The American Recovery and Reinvestment Act (ARRA) provided $1.1 billion for comparative effectiveness research.The Federal Coordinating Council for Comparative Effectiveness Research (FCCCER) aims to support healthcare policy decision makers by generating research that involves large scale pragmatic trials, patient databases and development of new quantitative methodologies.
- HTA is a process of evaluating the consequences of a new healthcare technology, as compared with products that are already available on the market. It summarizes information about the medical, social, economic and ethical issues related to the use of a health technology in a systematic, transparent, unbiased, robust manner. In order to generate this often sophisticated evidence, payers delegate the assessment to experts. Governments in most developed countries created HTA agencies, that have the expertise and that can act as independent stakeholders, not influenced by economic or political considerations.

The Value assessment by payers

Payers are concerned about the Value of the medicine in order to contain drug expenditure and invest in products that can create best health outcomes [15]. In this endeavour they need to assess the uncertainty about the drug's potential health benefits, as well as the potential costs related to funding it.

The process of assessing the Value for money of a medicine is broadly a four-step assessment, although not all payers go through the four steps described below.

1. Comparative efficacy from clinical trials (as compared to alternative treatments for the same condition): It aims at comparing two drugs in clinical trials and measuring the benefit of one over the other. The clinical trial design, the inclusion/exclusion criteria, the randomization procedure etc. may compromise the quality and reliability of the comparison and raise doubts for the payer on the actual effect size of the benefit.

2. Comparative effectiveness from real-life data on use of the medicine: If added benefit is observed in clinical trials, there are three potential obstacles for acknowledging the benefit in real life (effectiveness). The effect size of the additional benefit in clinical trial, the transferability across jurisdictions, and the transferability from a clinical trial model to real life; these three specific uncertainties are addressed at least qualitatively and ideally quantitatively. Some countries stop their assessment at this phase. If a medicine doesn't show significant benefit after these two steps, the Value will be considered equal or lower than that of the comparator treatment. In this situation, no premium price can be granted. However, if the benefit is shown, Value for money can be further assessed by comparing the extra benefits to the extra costs of the new medicine.

3. Cost effectiveness: This methodology compares the effectiveness benefit against the cost consequences (cost per Life Year Saved, per Quality Adjusted Life Year – QALY, per success, per relapse avoided etc.). Cost per QALY seems to have been increasingly adopted over the recent years in most HTA organization. As resources are limited

> **Box 3. Importance of affordability**
>
> - In the US, payers pay for some oncology products $ 80,0000 to increase life expectancy by 1.2 months. Then by extrapolation, survival of 1 year would be valued at $ 800,000. In the US, 550,000 patients die from cancer annually. If new drugs are developed that extend life by one year, $ 440 Billion would be needed to purchase these drugs for all patients. It is obviously unaffordable even for the richest country and unlikely to be affordable for any country.
> - Therefore, it seems that beyond assessing what is the Value of (additional health benefit) a new medicine, we need to be concerned about what is the affordability of the payer to fund this new medicine.

whenever a new intervention is introduced, the new one will displace the other available intervention (opportunity cost). It is important to consider if this opportunity is going to be at least as cost-effective as the one it displaced. Although it remains quite theoretical, as the effectiveness of intervention is often unknown at launch it is commonly considered rational to set a threshold for the incremental cost-effectiveness ratio (ICER) per QALY that represents the reference for available interventions that may be displaced.

4. Budget impact. This stage determines if the intervention is affordable in the current budget and if not, what is the additional budget needed to reimburse this new drug or what actions should be undertaken to make it affordable. Some countries do not consider budget impact as they believe it is redundant with the efficiency assessment, as the ICER threshold is expected to reflect/be adjusted on the affordability. This remains debatable (see Box 3).

Following Value assessment, the payers may wish to estimate what is the right price for the medicine in question. In general, four pricing models have been used by the pharmaceutical industry globally:

- Value based pricing. "It sets selling prices on the perceived value to the costumer, rather than on the actual cost of the product, the market price, competitors prices, or the historical price";
- Cost plus pricing. "One first calculates the cost of the product, then includes an additional amount to represent profit";
- Price benchmarking. "By observing the quality/value of products of other businesses, a company is able to use price benchmarking to determine a price for their products in relation to where they think they stand amongst the competition";
- Mixed model pricing.
- Pharmaceutical industry in the West currently uses a Mixed model that combines Value based pricing and benchmarking. In the institutionalized healthcare payer settings, Value based pricing is currently considered to be the most promising model, but the methodology is only emerging and it remains to be seen if it will be implemented successfully.

The link between HTA and Pricing & Reimbursement conditions

Negative HTA recommendation on use of a medicine translates into sub-optimal MA in various ways. The impact on price can be through direct reduction of the price by the payer, price-volume agreements or co-payments (Germany). The impact on reimbursement is by reducing the maximum percentage of reimbursement (France).

- Further, restrictions can be applied on the scope of prescription of a drug. Partial restriction consists in defining a population of patients or indication that is narrowed as compared to the Marketing Authorization of a drug. Full restriction means that a drug will not be included in formularies or in guidelines (Canada, UK). Pre-authorization of prescription by the payer or a specialist medical centre for a medicine are other means of ensuring that the drug is only prescribed to patients strictly defined by the payer. Finally, Market Access Agreements discussed in section 1.7 are confidential discount between the manufacturers and the payers that aim at obscuring the real list price or contracts allowing a temporary premium price until stronger evidence over drug's effectiveness or safety is developed.

Non-HTA tools that affect pricing

HTA is a laborious process and it's often unclear how to link its results to the price of a medicine. Reference pricing is a benchmarking model of setting prices of medicines by comparing them to the existing prices of the same medicine in other countries or by comparing them to prices of existing medicines in the same therapeutic area or with a similar mechanism of action in the same country.

External Reference Pricing

External Reference Pricing (ERP) (also referred to as "External Price Referencing", "International Price Benchmark", "External Price Benchmark", "External Price Linkage" or else "International Price Linkage") has rapidly become a widespread cost-containment tool put to use by the European countries for their pricing purposes, as well as by other countries such as Brazil, Jordan, South Africa, Japan, Turkey, Canada and Australia who refer to the European drug prices in order to establish their own [16].

The WHO Collaborating Centre for Pricing and Reimbursement Policies defines ERP as "the practice of using the price(s) of a medicine in one or several countries in order to derive a benchmark or reference price for the purposes of setting or negotiating the price of the product in a given country" [17]. Consequently, the change of price for a given product in one country affects the price in other countries. The use of ERP whether as a chief tool or as a supportive method to determine the price for new drugs entering the market in a vast majority of countries is supervised by health authorities within a pre-set legal framework.

E.g. in France, ERP methods are agreed within a framework agreement between the Healthcare Products Pricing Committee and the pharmaceutical companies. A similar framework agreement has been co-signed in Ireland between the Irish Pharmaceutical Healthcare Association Ltd and the Department of health and Healthcare Executives.

Altogether, ERP methods and rulings are outlined with contrasting levels of accuracy within the national pricing regulations depending on the countries and the level of priority devoted to this tool. Portugal and Austria are good examples of countries in which the legislation provides ample details on the use of ERP. German and Estonian laws provide much less guidance on the matter.

On one extreme, Luxembourg resorts to ERP to determine the price of all new marketed drugs. However, ERP is more often applied only to specific groups of medicines such as those publicly reimbursed, prescription-only medicines or else innovative products. As a matter of fact, many countries (Austria, Croatia, Czech Republic, Finland, Ireland, Italy, Latvia, Lithuania, Malta, Poland, Slovakia, Slovenia and Switzerland) apply ERP solely for publicly reimbursed medicines. Estonia, France and Germany resort to ERP in the case of innovative and publicly reimbursed medicines only.

Internal Reference Pricing

Benchmarking prices of existing medicines in the same therapeutic area or with a similar mechanism of action in the same country is used by some countries to set prices of new drugs. E.g. in Germany, when no additional benefit has been established in the HTA of a newly approved medicine, it is allocated to a reference price group with pharmacologically and therapeutically comparable pharmaceuticals. All pharmaceuticals in this group will have the same price so called 'jumbo groups'. In many European countries, an internal reference pricing system is in place for reimbursed generics, that is all products that contain the same off-patent molecule are priced at the same level [16].

.7 Market Access Agreements

Definition

High cost of novel treatments is a common cause of negative or restricted reimbursement decisions by healthcare payers. Such decisions can reduce or even eliminate MA for new products. This reflects on patient's access to those treatments and also on the revenue of the manufacturers. Poor patients' access results in political pressure on the payers and other healthcare authorities. Reduced revenue reflects on the company management and the shareholders. Therefore, both the payers and the industry seek compromise in achieving MA for novel products.

The outcome of such negotiations can be called Market Access Agreements (MAA). MAA can be defined as "an agreement between two or more parties, who agree on the terms and conditions under which a product will get access to the market". MAA specify, often in a confidential manner, the conditions under which a concerned treatment will be priced and reimbursed in a given population of patients.

To date, there is a confusion surrounding the exact definition of MAA and there is no commonly agreed definition for MAA. In fact, a number of definitions can be found in the literature. MAA are often referred to as risk sharing agreements, despite the lack of risk sharing in most of them. Consultants call them innovative contracting, or Managed Entry Agreements while in UK a new terminology was adopted by the Department of Health (DoH) Patient Access Scheme (PAS). Risk sharing, cost sharing and Payment for Performance (P4P), are often put in the same basket and called risk sharing agreements, whereas in reality, there are some structural differences [18].

Taxonomy

To simplify the nomenclature and taxonomy, MAA can be generally grouped into financial (Commercial Agreements, CA) or outcomes-based (P4P or Coverage with Evidence Development – CED) [19]:

- Financial agreements are CA between two or more parties entering into a deal for goods acquisition;
- Outcome-based agreements are part of an insurance or warranty facility. The payer agrees to a price under the insurance that the product will deliver a predefined health outcome in a given patient. This regroups two kinds of MAA: P4P and CED.

These two types of MAAs are subdivided in two categories, MAA at the population level (certain types of CA, such as price-volume agreements, CED) and MAA at the individual patient level (certain types of CA, such as price cap per patient, free drug supply after a pre-defined treatment duration etc., P4P).

P4P are agreed by payers to avoid expenditure on treating patients who do not respond to a drug and who cannot be identified *ex ante*, by permanently linking the payment to drug's performance in individual patients. P4P is set to pay only for patients who achieve a pre-specified response to a drug.

In contrast, CED are temporary MAA where the payers agree to finance the new technology as a part of a well-designed study, in order to generate in real-life evidence that will enable final price and reimbursement decisions. Such evidence may not be available at the time of drug launch, because data from clinical trials does not reflect the use, health outcome, dosage or duration of treatment in real-life, actual targeted patient population or the impact of the medicine in question on the use of other healthcare resources.

Finally, MAA can be a mix of two types of agreements, e.g., a simple price discount (CA) is often an element of P4P.

The future

CA and P4P ensure drug cost reductions to payers while maintaining high list prices. The importance of high list prices for the industry pertains from the use of External Reference Pricing globally. Therefore, maintaining high visible prices in the major pharmaceutical markets can help manufacturers ensure high prices in countries that use those countries to set prices of new drugs. The introduction of differential pricing that depends e.g. on the country GDP/capita instead of ERP or a combination of both could accelerate disappearance of CA and P4P because it will no longer make sense to strive for high list prices while the real prices are lower. Indeed, P4P have been documented to be costly and burdensome to implement by healthcare providers, payers and the manufacturers. However, in Europe and elsewhere the resistance to differential pricing is fuelled by parallel trade which may negatively impact manufacturers' revenue and the availability of drugs in countries where they are sold at a lower price.

- In the future, the complex and burdensome P4P will likely be replaced by CA when payers need to reduce the cost or by CED when they wish to reduce uncertainty about a drug's performance.

References

1. Introduction to Market Access in Trade in Goods in the WTO, WTO e-learning. Available at https://ecampus.wto.org/admin/files/Course_385/Module_1578/ModuleDocuments/MA-L1-R1-E.pdf (last accessed September 2016)
2. Olcay M, Laing R. Pharmaceutical tariffs: what is their effect on prices, protection of local industry, and revenue generation: Commission on Intellectual Property Rights, Innovation and public health. May 2005. Available at http://www.who.int/intellectualproperty/studies/TariffsOnEssentialMedicines.pdf?ua=1 (last accessed September 2016)
3. European Commission. Pharmaceuticals Sector Fiche. Brussels 16.12.2011
4. Tracy K, Guzman D, Burton M. Treatment Process and Participant Characteristic Predictors of Substance Use Outcome in Mentorship for Addiction Problems (MAP). *J Alcohol Drug Depend* 2014; 2: 171
5. Squires D, Anderson C. U.S. health care from a global perspective: spending, use of services, prices, and health in 13 countries. *Issue Brief (Commonw Fund)* 2015; 15: 1-15
6. European Commission. Procedures for evaluating medicinal products and granting marketing authorisation. Available at http://ec.europa.eu/health/authorisation-procedures_en.htm (last accessed September 2016)
7. Menger C. Principles of Economics. Auburn, Ala: Ludwig von Mises Institute, 2007
8. Desogus C. Antitrust issues in the European pharmaceutical market: an economic analysis of recent cases on parallel trade. Available at https://www.upf.edu/cres/_pdf/wp60_desogus.pdf (last accessed September 2016)
9. Woolhandler S, Himmelstein DU. Competition in a publicly funded healthcare system. *BMJ* 2007; 335: 1126-9
10. Kumar A, Juluru K, Thimmaraju P et al. Pharmaceutical market access in emerging markets: concepts, components, and future. *Journal of Market Access & Health Policy* 2014; 2: 25302
11. Rémuzat C, Toumi M, Falissard B. New drug regulations in France: what are the impacts on market access? Part 2 - impacts on market access and impacts for the pharmaceutical industry. *Journal of Market Access & Health Policy* 2013; 1: 20892
12. Mittendorf T, Theidel U. Market Access Fundamentals in Germany: AMNOG's Decisions Yield Valuable Insights. *HTA Quarterly* Fall 2014. Available at

http://www.xcenda.com/Insights-Library/HTA-Quarterly-Archive-Insights-to-Bridge-Science-and-Policy/HTA-Quarterly-Fall-2014/Market-Access-Fundamentals-in-Germany-AMNOGs-Decisions-Yield-Valuable-Insights-/ (last accessed September 2016)

13. Tolley, K. Pharmaceutical market access and the challenges of health technology assessment in the United Kingdom. *Drug Dev Res* 2010; 71: 478-84

14. Ess SM, Schneeweiss S, Szucs TD. European Healthcare Policies for Controlling Drug Expenditure, *Pharmacoeconomics* 2003; 21: 89-103

15. New Approaches to Gaining MA for Pharmaceuticals: Pricing & Reimbursement, Policy Development, and the Role of HTAs. Business Insights Limited, 2010

16. Ruggeri K, Nolte E. Pharmaceutical pricing The use of external reference pricing. RAND Corporation, 2013 available at http://www.rand.org/content/dam/rand/pubs/research_reports/RR200/RR240/RAND_RR240.pdf (last accessed September 2016)

17. Toumi M, Remuzat C, Vataire AL, et al. External reference pricing of medicinal products: simulation-based considerations for cross-country coordination. European Commission, 2014. Available at http://ec.europa.eu/health/healthcare/docs/erp_reimbursement_medicinal_products_en.pdf (last accessed September 2016)

18. Toumi M, Michel M. Define Access Agreements. PMlive, 2011. Available at http://www.pmlive.com/pharma_news/define_access_agreements_283271# (last accessed September 2016)

19. Jarosławski S, Toumi M. Market access agreements for pharmaceuticals in Europe: diversity of approaches and underlying concepts. *BMC Health Serv Res* 2011; 11: 259

1.9 **To know more**

- Global Trade Negotiations Home Page. Available at http://www.cid.harvard.edu/cidtrade/issues/marketaccess.html (last accessed September 2016)
- Kristensen FB, Sigmund H. Health Technology Assessment Handbook. Copenhagen: Danish Centre for Health Technology Assessment, National Board of Health, 2007
- Surveying, Assessing and Analysing the Pharmaceutical Sector in the 25 EU Member States. Commissioned by European Commission – DG Competition, 2006. Available at http://ec.europa.eu/competition/mergers/studies_reports/oebig.pdf (last accessed September 2016)
- Garattini L, Cornago D, De Compadri P. Pricing and reimbursement of in-patent drugs in seven European countries: A comparative analysis. *Health Policy* 2007; 82: 330-9
- Market access for Pharma: pulling in the same direction? – a UK perspective from Alan Crofts. Available at http://www.thepharmaletter.com/file/79052/market-

access-for-pharma-pulling-in-the-same-direction-a-uk-perspective-from-alan-crofts.html (last accessed September 2016)
- Robinson SW. Market Access – The Definition Depends on the Viewpoint. Evidence Matters 2010; 16. Available at http://www.paramountcommunication.com/ubc/pdf/01_Market_Access_The_Definition.pdf (last accessed September 2016)
- Claxton K, Briggs A, Buxton MJ, et al. Value based pricing for NHS drugs: an opportunity not to be missed. *BMJ* 2008; 336: 251-4
- Sackett DL, Rosenberg WM, Gray JA et al. Evidence based medicine: what it is and what it isn't. *BMJ* 1996; 312: 71-2
- Menger C. Principles of Economics, translated by J. Dingwall and B. F. Hoselitz, Glencoe, IL: Free Press, 1950 [original 1871]

Market Access in Asian countries

Kally Wong

"Emerging Markets" is a term first employed by Antoine van Agtmael, an investment officer with the International Financial Corporation (IFC—part of World Bank Group) in 1981. He was referring to a new perspective on the potential of developing countries, with their total capitalization projected to reach US$ 5 trillion in a 25-year period. In 1986, IFC promoted the Emerging Market Growth Fund, the first mutual fund of its kind for developing countries [1]. In 2003, Goldman Sachs put the concept of BRIC countries (Brazil, Russia, India, and China) under the spotlight in global investment markets. They represent countries within emerging markets which are broadly defined as developing markets that experienced and anticipate a fast rate of economic growth. However, this "fast rate" is a relative concept, and it is set against a comparison with those of the developed western countries, and Japan.

As the definition of "emerging markets" lies in their rate of growth rather than other absolute financial indicators such as the various forms of Gross Domestic Products (GDPs), South Korea is included in the category of "emerging markets" in Asia for the fact that its rate of growth is comparable at the level of other countries in that group of classification, albeit the fact that South Korea has an advanced economic and business environment, and the fact that it also has a health insurance system that is increasingly served as a reference for other East Asian countries.

Thus, while the focus of this chapter is on market access for emerging markets in Asia, the definition for the category is by virtue of the speed of their growing spending on healthcare services. To illustrate the different types of development, three countries from the basket of "emerging markets" are chosen for this chapter: China, Thailand, and South Korea.

The GDP growth rate for these three markets has been phenomenal since the 1990s, with China being the exemplar of them all. China has maintained an annual GDP growth rate above 8% since the year 2000, and surpassed Japan as the second biggest economy in 2010. The recent forecast for economic growth in China is that it would still stay at the high level of 7% in 2015. The living standard of a large number of people has been elevated, and a new middle class has started to emerge. People are growing to inspire for a quality healthcare service as they get more affluence. Health outcomes and costs in Asian emerging markets in 2014 are reported in Table 1.

Yet, a common trait among the emerging markets in Asia is that within each market there is a large income disparity, with low income groups being the majority of the total population. Most are also facing the challenge of limited resources in developing a nationwide healthcare infrastructure. It is against this background that the latest healthcare policies for emerging markets in Asia are formulating.

Country	GDP per capita (US$) 2013	Health spending per head (US$)	Total expenditure on health as % of GDP 2013	Health spending rank[2]	Health outcomes rank[2]
Japan[1]	38,634	4,714	10.3	153	166
Singapore[1]	55,182	2,538	4.6	145	165
South Korea	25,977	1,834	7.8	137	152
China	6,807	337	5.6	86	120
Vietnam	1,911	116	6.0	51	110
Thailand	5,779	214	4.6	67	104
Malaysia	10,538	417	4.0	94	80
Indonesia	3,475	106	3.1	48	75
Cambodia	1,007	51	7.5	28	62
Philippines	2,765	119	4.4	52	61
Pakistan	1,275	34	3.0	15	55
India	1,498	62	4.0	33	52

Table 1. Health outcomes and costs in Asian emerging markets, 2014 [2-4]
[1] Japan and Singapore are not considered as Asian emerging markets
[2] Among 166 countries comparison (166 = highest)

2.1 Overview on the Healthcare Systems and Healthcare Policies

In general, governments of the emerging markets in Asia do recognize the importance of addressing the issue of public healthcare. However, for any initiatives to improve the quality of healthcare services and related facilities, they must also find ways to ensure an equal access to those services. Addressing this problem effectively involves the development of some type of health insurance system. This, in turn, have to take into a number of considerations; viz., who should be given the reimbursement, what should be the level of coverage in reimbursement, what types of healthcare provisions should be reimbursed; and at a more macro level of consideration, how the healthcare system should be financed, how much of the government resources should be allocated on healthcare, etc.

Malaysia, Hong Kong, Vietnam, Singapore, and China are examples of a private sector driven market. Due to different economic and political structures, the concept of universal healthcare coverage in Asia is perceived rather differently from Western countries. Asian healthcare systems are characterized by high co-payment with only a limited range of reimbursements.

South Korea

South Korea is a growth model for how a healthcare system in Asia can evolve under an optimal situation. In the 1960s, the annual income per head in South Korea was US$ 87, which was on a par with the poorest parts of Africa and only two-third of the GDPs of the Philippines. South Korea was then one of the poorest countries in the world. In 1962, the government implemented its first Five-Year Economic Development Plan. At that time, the GDP was barely US$ 2.7 billion. Yet, since the introduction of the first economic development plan, it was able to maintain an average annual growth rate of 8% between 1960s and 1980s. Even though this rate started to dip after three decades of strong growth, it was still at 6.5% by 1989; a very strong growth by most measures. The recent GDP growth rate for 2013 was 3%, but it already has a GDP of US$ 1.305 trillion, compared with a GDP barely US$ 2.7 billion in 1962 and a GDP of US$ 230 billion in 1989 [3].

The first social insurance scheme (Employee Scheme) was introduced in South Korea in 1977 which was exclusively for companies hiring at least 500 employees. It was catered for the needs of Chaebol, a South Korea type of business conglomerates. The insurance scheme aimed to provide stability in the workforce. The tens of thousands of teachers, students, and people who worked in small business would not benefit from any healthcare coverage under this first scheme.

The situation was improved in 1980, when the Social Health Insurance (SHI) was implemented. This new scheme provided healthcare coverage for employees in small business and schools. Nine years later, in 1989, the first National Health Insurance (NHI) was launched. In 2006, the South Korean government started to use evidence based assessment on reimbursement decisions for new medical technologies applications (including diagnostics, surgical procedures, and devices). As of 2012, 7,350 out of 8,067 medical services are covered in reimbursements. Effectively, 96% of total population, which is estimated to have 49 million people in 2014 [5], have health insurance coverage. At present, South Korea is regarded to have the most advanced health technology assessment in Asia.

South Korea achieved a universal healthcare system within a very short time. Its development projects the potentials for future healthcare systems for low and middle income Asian countries. The National Health Insurance in South Korea is characterized by a comparatively small amount of public contribution for a basic coverage of healthcare services for almost the whole population. In addition, South Korea is one of the few countries in the world managing their health insurance at a surplus. To illustrate how the system works, NHI received a revenue of Won 47.2 trillion (US$ 42.48 billion) in 2013, with 82.7% of it came from insurance premium, 10.2% from government subsidies, and 7% from tobacco consumption tax. After deducting an expenditure of Won 41.3 trillion (US$ 37.17 billion), Korean government recorded Won 5.9 trillion (US$ 5.31 billion) surplus in 2013.

Effectively, the South Korea government has established a well-financed healthcare system. People are used to paying out-of-pocket for a better quality of healthcare services. This system of financing has the significant advantage of reducing the financial burden on the government in providing healthcare services.

China

Compared with the health insurance and healthcare system in South Korea, China represents a different stage of development. Along with its growth of the economy, China seems to be moving in the direction of a universal healthcare as well. Chinese government has been increasing the access to medical services and improving the efficiency of the healthcare system in the past 25 years. Certainly it would take time to have a complete roll-out of a universal healthcare for a country with the geographical and population size of China. On the other hand, the huge gap in the quality of health services that existed in the different parts of the country does seem to be gradually narrowing.

Theoretically, the healthcare system in China is meant to be based on the principle of socialism. Yet, it has been operating with a hybrid of occupational welfare and free market-mechanism since the 1990s. After the reform initiated in the 1980s, the economy was first taken-off in the priority cities, which were the capital city of Beijing, and the two coastal cities of Shanghai and Guangzhou. Furthermore, urbanization of the coastal cities was encouraged and indeed, prevalent. Initially, Chinese healthcare insurance coverage were limited to certain groups of people in the country, these were senior ranking government officials, veteran soldiers of the 1927-1950 civil war and those people who have made "special contributions to the nation". These restricted groups of people benefited under the Government Insurance Scheme (GIS). Under another scheme, the Labor Insurance Scheme (LIS), minimal medical allowance was available for those who worked in state enterprises. For those who lived in rural area, medical allowance was almost non-existence. Access to basic medical services for the rural population was through "barefoot doctors" in the villages, who were "doctors with minimal training in primary healthcare". The majority of Chinese was paying out-of-pocket for their medical expenses at that time.

Yet, with social and economic changes resulted from the economic reform, many people came to expect being able to enjoy certain degree of healthcare benefits in the better-off cities. As expected would be the case when policies could not catch up with social changes, government subsidies for hospitals became inadequate with the raise in public healthcare expenditure which was increasingly borne by healthcare institutions themselves. Chinese government began to experience the pressure of allocating more resources to support the medical institutions.

In 1998, the first Urban Basic Health Insurance Scheme (UBHIS)/(UEBMI) (Note: the English abbreviation of this Urban Health Insurance Scheme has two different versions, depending on which government body uses the term) was implemented and administered by local governments. Employees who lived in urban areas became entitled to healthcare benefits. The percentage of contributions by employees and employers varies across provinces, but it was estimated that 39% of the total urban residents were benefited from this change of policy.

Following the trend of its economic policy, China also saw a raise in the level of "privatization" as well as decentralization of the government role in the healthcare provision between 1978 and 1999. Hospitals were shifted to run on a self-balance budget. Central government has also transferred the responsibility of healthcare provision to local governments at the provincial and municipal level. Source of healthcare funding has changed from exclusively central government to mostly local governments through local taxation.

The change at this period of time also resulted in the significant role local governments play in market access. Starting from that period, local governments were forced to operate healthcare as a service industry to cover their expenses.

In 2003, the healthcare coverage extended to a wider population. Local government at the county level introduced the New Rural Cooperative Medical Scheme (NRCMS) for people who lived in the rural areas. It was the first time that a limited reimbursement coverage was available to rural residents, although they accounted for the majority of total population at the time. The estimation was that about 70% people lived in rural area in 2000, and 50% in 2012 [6]. However, even with this change of policy, rural residents still had difficulties in accessing to medical services. There were simply not much medical facilities or institutions available because of the long deprived resources in the healthcare infrastructure in the countryside. Hospitals were mostly located in medium and large cities, or Tier II and Tier I cities using the Chinese government's definition. Rural residents had to travel a long way to seek medical treatment. The national health insurance system was very much in the early stage of development in practice. In addition, medical treatments were far too expensive for most rural residents. An estimated 87% of rural patients still had to pay the full cost of medical treatment out-of-pocket by the late 2000s. The rural population was also the group of population that had the lowest income by far.

The Urban Residents Basic Medical Insurance (URBMI) was the third major health insurance scheme in China. It was enacted in 2005 with the aim to cover those urban residents who were not covered in UBHIS, and they could obtain reimbursement of at least 50% of the basic medical fees.

In the Medical Reform of 2009-2012, the government set a primary goal of providing a nationwide basic medical coverage. They aimed to change the healthcare service so that it would be affordable and accessible for all, under some form of coverage. In 2013, the central government envisioned the notion of a "Healthy China 2020", which means that the aim is to have a healthcare system of universal coverage by then.

Throughout the time, it is true to say that the central government has attempted to make healthcare service available to a wider public. The way the Central government carried this out was by grasping price control on standard diagnostics tests, routine pharmaceutical products and routine surgeries, etc. A central government department, the National Development and Reform Commission (NDRC), was assigned to formulate drug pricing policies. There was some degree of flexibility on price setting in a few special circumstances. It allowed local healthcare facilities to make profit on advanced technology, new drugs and new tests with independent pricing. Patents drugs were given flexibility to set their level of pricing. However, this arrangement has been put under scrutiny in the Medical Reform between 2009 and 2012. As a result, originators of the off-patent drugs and the me-too patent drugs lost the privilege of free price setting. They are now being targeted for government price control.

Thailand

Thailand represents another model of health insurance and healthcare system in Asia. Unlike South Korea and China, the universal healthcare coverage was not driven by a fast economic growth this time.

Thailand is one of the few low to middle income Asian emerging markets which implemented universal healthcare (called Universal Coverage Scheme—UCS) as early as in 2002. Thailand also has the most extensive coverage of WHO recommended essential drugs in their National List Essential Medicine (NLED). According to the World Bank, it is estimated 99.5% of Thai people are under some forms of healthcare coverage in 2014. In that respect, Thailand has made a significant achievement on its healthcare in the past 30 years. The level of success is reflected through its record of curbing the incidences of HIV/AIDS and reducing child mortality rate. The death rate due to HIV/ AIDS was 86.2 per 100,000 population in 2000, and it was dropped to 31.0 per 100,000 population by 2012. Similarly, the under-five child mortality rate was 37 per 1,000 live births in 1990, and it was dropped to 13 per 1,000 live births in 2013 [7].

Despite the significant strife it made in its healthcare structure, there remain some issues within the system that needs to be addressed. One concern is the lacking of healthcare facilities in the rural area, especially in North Eastern region. This area is mainly agrarian in nature, and is considered poorer than other areas. Doctor-to-patient ratio, at 3 doctors per 10,000 patients, is relatively low. Many Thais also could not afford the good quality healthcare services which are mostly available in the private sector.

The underlying problem for continuing improvement on the healthcare structure in Thailand is the already constrained public finances, as well as uncertainties in the political environment for the past 8 years.

Basically, the healthcare structure of Thailand contains three major types of health insurance scheme, and they are managed by three different government departments. The first health insurance scheme was designed for civil servants and their family members as a fringe benefit working for the government. It is called the Civil Servants Medical Benefits Scheme (CSMBS) and it was in place since 1978. This scheme is fully funded through part of the general taxation. Its management is under the Comptroller's General Department in the Ministry of Finance. It is estimated that 7 million people came under the coverage of CSMBS. As of 2008, the government implemented cost containment measures on pharmaceutical products, and that had some effect on CSMBS. For example, there is no longer free-pricing on original products, but these products are now set at the median price based on international reference pricing (for products on the National List of Essential Drugs—NLED). Reimbursement coverage on multinational pharmaceutical products has also been cut down under CSMBS.

After the release of the Draft of the Social Security Act 1990, people working in the private sector became benefited from the Social Security Scheme (SSS) and have insurance against circumstances of illness, accident, physical disability, child delivery, old age, child assistance, unemployment and death not related to the work duties [8]. The SSS is a compulsory insurance scheme for people who work for private companies and its funding is contributed by employees, employers and the government. This insurance scheme is run by the Social Security Office and provided health coverage to 11 million people. Together, CSMBS and SSS provided health coverage to about 22% of the total population.

UCS is the most recent health insurance scheme introduced. Its coverage extends to 47 million people, which is almost 79% of the total population in Thailand. UCS is managed by the National Health Security Office (NHSO). The scheme was initiated by the ruling government at that time, which was Thai Rak Thai (TRT). Registered members of this scheme are able to receive treatment with a co-payment of just 30 bahts (US$ 0.9). It provides healthcare coverage to those who are not covered in CSMBS or SSS. It also extends the healthcare coverage to those who were originally covered under a more restricted Medical Welfare Scheme for the poor. UCS was rolled out nationwide with a testing period of six months in selected cities. Unlike China and South Korea, the universal healthcare scheme in Thailand was introduced in the absence of a fast-growing economy, and became a financial burden on Thailand's public healthcare expenditure. As a result of its implementation, public healthcare spending increased from 66 billion bahts in 2001 (US$ 2 billion) to 169.8 billion bahts (US$ 5.15 billion) in 2008. The recent figure on public spending in healthcare in 2013 was 253 billion bahts (US$ 7.67 billion) [9].

After the Thai Rak Thai government, there have been two military coups since, in 2007 and 2014. These military coups did not put a halt on the ballooning healthcare cost though. UCS was modified in 2008 by the interim military government and it put forward the 30-baht co-payment on an even more generous ground. Patients could pay the

Country	2005	2006	2007	2008	2009	2010	2011	2012	2013
Japan[1]	8.2	8.2	8.2	8.6	9.5	9.6	10.1	10.3	10.3
Singapore[1]	3.7	3.6	3.4	3.9	4.3	3.9	3.9	4.2	4.6
South Korea	5.7	6.1	6.4	6.6	7.2	7.3	7.4	7.6	7.8
China	4.7	4.6	4.4	4.6	5.1	5.0	5.1	5.4	5.6
Vietnam	5.4	6.0	6.5	5.5	6.0	6.4	6.2	6.0	6.0
Thailand	3.5	3.5	3.6	3.9	4.1	3.8	4.1	4.5	4.6
Malaysia	3.3	3.7	3.6	3.5	4.0	4.0	3.9	4.0	4.0
Indonesia	2.8	2.9	3.1	2.8	2.8	2.9	2.9	3.0	3.1
Cambodia	5.8	4.2	3.5	5.5	6.3	5.8	5.6	7.3	7.5
Philippines	3.9	4.0	3.9	3.9	4.3	4.2	4.3	4.4	4.4
Pakistan	2.8	2.8	3.2	3.7	3.6	3.4	2.9	3.0	3.0
India	4.3	4.1	3.9	4.0	4.1	3.8	3.8	3.8	4.0

Table 2. Total expenditure on health as percentage of Gross Domestic Product 2005-2013 [4]
[1] Japan and Singapore are not considered as Asian emerging markets

30 bahts on a voluntary basis, and medical treatments were offered almost free to the public.

The 30-baht co-payment method was revamped in 2012 by the Puea Thai Party, which was a metamorphosis of the Thai Rat Thai Party earlier. Patients had to pay the 30-baht consultation fee again.

As this extensive universal healthcare scheme is proving to be very popular among the low income groups, it is unlikely that any government is going to reverse this public health policy any time soon. The challenge for the present and future governments in Thailand is how to address the mounting healthcare spending brought by a universal health scheme. The government at present is actively implementing a number of cost containment measures, including curbing the surging spending on pharmaceutical products under CSMBS. Generic prescriptions and single pricing are enforced. Economic assessment on drug prices has been carried out for pharmaceutical products in NLED. The Health Intervention and Technology Assessment Program (HITAP) was introduced in 2006. The National Health Technology Assessment (HTA) guidelines and database were released in 2007 and they were further updated in 2012. In 2015, NHSO decided to control the healthcare spending further by freezing hospital subsidies and lowering the budget for universal healthcare.

Total expenditure on health as percentage of Gross Domestic Product 2005-2013 is reported in Table 2.

2.2 Recent Healthcare Policies

The economic growth is expected to remain positive for South Korea for the near future. The real GDP growth in 2014 was recorded as 3.4% in South Korea and 7.4% in China.

Thailand

Thailand is still anticipating a stagnant economy due to the lack of confidence in consumers and private business, and its real GDP growth in 2014 was 0.2%. However positive the economic prospect of the country is, these Asian governments share one thing in common: It is the uncertainties associated with the growing demand on healthcare resources and welfare spending. Overall speaking, health inequalities and accessibilities still remain the two key challenges for these emerging market governments. Further healthcare issues include an aging population and increasing prevalence of chronic diseases which are closely associated with the fast-changing environment. They include hypertension, diabetes, chronic obstructive pulmonary disease, etc. It would be imperative for any successful healthcare policy to be able to achieve a relatively sound healthcare structure while able to control the cost. This daunting aspect inevitably means that there would be on-going healthcare reforms.

Thailand is half way through its eleventh National Development Plan 2012-2016. In its recent healthcare policy, the priority is to improve the quality, the affordability and the accessibility of medical services for the entire population. The development of primary healthcare services in community healthcare centers is going to be paramount. Cost-containment measures on pharmaceutical products would continue. There is a strong debate on the integration of three health insurance schemes, with the basic underlying goal being able to harmonize the price and reimbursement packages of the three schemes. It is expected that discussions on the merging of the three health insurance schemes would go-on for at least sometime. At present, only the emergency service has been harmonized. Patients are now able to receive free treatment on emergency services in all the hospitals that is part of any of the three health insurance schemes.

However, if the uncertainties on political front persist, Thailand is unlikely to have any significant structural changes to its healthcare system in the near future.

South Korea

In South Korea, the government has increased welfare coverage for the elderly population through a new state pension plan for retirees aged 65 and above, regardless of their income. Health insurance contribution from the government seems ready to maintain at a level of 6.07%, compared with the average 10-12% insurance contribution in G8 countries for 2013. Furthermore, there is no sign of changes on the patient co-payment policy which remains at 36.6% in 2013. Compared with the average of 19.1% in OECD (Organization for Economic Cooperation and Development) countries, the South Korean co-payment policy seems ready to maintain at that relatively high level. To contain healthcare spending, the government has already widely implemented a list of measures, including the pharmacoeconomic assessment on reimbursement drug by Health Insurance Review & Assessment Service (HIRA), price-volume agreements, a positive reimbursement list and promote the prescription of generics. Currently, the government is also reviewing the use of global budget and reference pricing which might add on to its pharmaceutical products price containment measures.

China

Since the announcement of a large scale medical reform between 2009 and 2012, the Chinese government has directed its medical reform at different levels. In the recent policy address in April 2015, the National Health and Family Planning Commission (NHFPC) plans to increase the health insurance premium for the unemployed and the children in the urban area. At the same time, they are also directing more healthcare resources to the rural population. The government restated its target of having healthcare coverage for 95% of the population by 2015. To rectify the problem of the over-reliance of public hospitals on drug sales, thus causing over-prescription problems, the Chinese government has also introduced the policy of separating treatment consultations and drug dispensary in public hospitals, which is now under a pilot scheme in 34 cities. This new policy stipulates that doctors' remuneration would be improved and their performance would not be assessed solely based on the number of prescriptions given to patients and the number of patients treated. The size of Level III hospitals, which are the large general and specialist hospitals, would be restricted for "unreasonable" expansion. The number of Level I hospitals, which are small community hospitals in China, would also be increased based on demographic structure of the area. Part of the income from government lottery would be diverted financing healthcare for the elderly. Healthcare efficiency and healthcare cost containment remain on the top of government's agenda. In addition, drug prices in public hospitals are under review, the purchase of drugs in the Essential Drug List (EDL) at the provincial level using local tenders is encouraged. The decision of removing the retail price cap on low-cost products in National Essential Drug List has just been confirmed in May 2015 by the NDRC.

In view of the recent effort by the government in China to improve its healthcare quality and accessibility, the medical reform seems to be on track for a healthcare structure that would cover the whole country. When that is established, it would then have a genuine universal healthcare system. As there are frequent discrepancies in policies issued by the central government and their local implementation, the concern remains as to what extent the central government and local governments could align in the implementation of healthcare reforms consistently and uniformly.

Price and reimbursement tools in selected Asian emerging markets in 2014 are reported in Table 3.

	South Korea	China	Thailand	Taiwan[1]	Singapore[1]
Profit control		P/SI			
Reference pricing	FI	P/SI	FI	FI	UI
Price cuts, freezes, ceiling		FI	FI		
Discounts and rebate				FI	FI
Pricing negotiations	FI	FI	FI	FI	FI
Positive/negative list	FI	FI	FI	FI	
Pharmacoeconomics	FI	P/SI	FI	FI	FI
Generic name prescribing				FI	
Pharmacist substitution	P/SI		FI	FI	
Patient co-pays	FI	FI	FI	FI	FI
Price-volume agreement	FI			FI	
Risk sharing agreement	P/SI				

Table 3. Price and reimbursement tools in selected Asian emerging markets in 2014
[1] Not categorized as an emerging market in Asia
FI = Fully implemented; P/SI = Partially/Soon to-be implemented; UI = Unlikely to implement

3 Pathways of Market Access

South Korea

Considering from the perspective of market access for pharmaceutical products, South Korea is unique in a number of aspects. Specifically, the market has:

- a high health insurance coverage (96% of total population in 2013);
- a large number of reimbursable drugs (about 17,000 in 2014);
- a high usage of original drugs (35.4% market share in value in 2014);
- a low generic substitution by pharmacists (1% in 2014);
- a very well-established IT systems tracking the prescription activities and reviewing the reimbursement benefits;
- a declining importance of sales detailing by medical representatives due to the dual punishing approach for both physicians and the pharmaceutical company against illegal rebate starting from 2010; and
- fewer new products launched (e.g. only half of the 45 newest oncology drugs have been launched in South Korea between 2009 and 2014).

Health insurance is compulsory by law. Ministry Of Health, Welfare and Family Affairs (MOHWFA) is responsible for the policy formulation on healthcare matters, including the health insurance program. National Health Insurance Corporation is the central government body to implement and manage the national health insurance service. Health Insurance Review Agency was established in 2000 after the government reformed the health insurance structure.

HIRA is the agency for healthcare benefit management as well as review and assessment in the price and reimbursement process. They use an evidence-based assessment. They conduct pharmaco-economic evaluation and assessment on the appropriateness of benefits inclusion of the new drug with the parameter of national reimbursement (Positive List System). The assessment is measured against cost-effectiveness and substitutability of the drug. HIRA Assessment Committee decides if the new drug should be included as a covered benefit. For the new health technology, the eligible case would be given a Resource-Based Relative Value (RBRV) score for reimbursement or an upper limit for the price. The process, starting from the submission of drug assessment application to the release of decision by MOHWFA, would take approximately 360 working days.

To attain the goal of quality improvement and cost control, HIRA provides a real-time drug safety information for medical institutions (Drug Utilization Review—DUR), and gives financial incentives to healthcare providers who manage to show a cost-effective treatment practice (Value Incentive Program—VIP). Looking at the past record of HIRA, the number of claims that need to be reviewed increased from 439 million in 2000 to 1,339 million in 2012.

The price of reimbursed drug is reviewed, and negotiated, by NHI. Several methods are used in this price setting process, such as Price-Volume Agreements (PVAs), and Rewards for Saving Drug Expenditure (RSDE), the latter replaced the Market-based Actual Transaction Pricing (MATP or ATP) in late 2014. According to the new NHI price negotiation guideline released on June 5, 2015, a new regulation will be implemented. Unless further negotiation is called for, the drug price for a new product would be 90% of the weighted average price (WAP) of comparable drugs if it is not an innovative product; 100% for orphan drugs and 95% for pediatric drugs. The introduction of generics drug will lead to 30% price-cut of the original drug. After more than 3 generics products launched in market, the price of generics and original drug will both be fixed and will keep at a level of 53.55% of the price of original product before its patent expired.

Likewise, according to the principle of Equal Maximum Price (EMP), biosimilar products and biologic products would keep their maximum price at 70% of the original brand. The South Korean government adopts a relatively open policy to encourage the development of the biosimilar market, including on its price setting. This is in response to the government vision of building their own capacity in exporting pharmaceutical products by 2020, more specifically in the areas of biosimilar.

The cost containment measures, which have been in place for almost a decade, was a result of the Drug Expenditure Rationalization Plan. It was first announced by MOHWFA in 2006. At the same year, the price of total 16,000 reimbursed drugs in 49 drug groups started being reviewed and the price of each drug was reassessed. The entire price review process was only completed in 2014 [10].

As a result of the process, the government has effectively achieved its goal in cost control on pharmaceutical products. Drug price in South Korea is approximately 44% of the average drug price of the OECD countries [11]. For the pharmaceutical industry, this "achievement" is rather debatable. The low drug price for new products raises business concerns as the worry is whether it would create a domino effect on the drug price of new products launched in other geographical markets. As a result, it seems that companies would tend to delay the launch of new products. At least, companies might put South Korea in a late order in the launch sequence. To encourage innovative products launch in the country, HIRA Review Committee has given fast-track reviews on new drug applications and speed up the reimbursement assessment. In the first half of 2015, there are 10 new drug applications and 8 of them were given fast track reviews. In addition to the fast track review for new innovative products, NHI gives an exemption on rare cancer and rare disease drugs from pharmacoeconomic evaluation. This is on top of the flexible score on incremental cost-effectiveness ratio (ICER) for anti-cancer treatment. The aim is to increase the acceptable optimal drug price for innovative drugs, and help to increase the number of new product launch in market [12].

South Korea contribution rate in National Health Insurance system and co-payment for in- and outpatients are reported in Tables 4 and 5.

Self-employed's monthly contribution is calculated by contribution score × value per points (Won 178 = US$ 0.159).

National Evidence based healthcare Collaborating Agency (NECA) is an independent government department set up in 2009 to facilitate the price and reimbursement process. It has two divisions; one is the Division Healthcare Technology Assessment Research. It responds to *ad hoc* requests from MOHWFA on reviewing the urgent listing of

	2009	2010	2011	2012	2013	2014	2015
Employee % of monthly wage	5.08	5.33	5.64	5.80	5.89	5.99	6.07
Self-employed[1] Value per point (KW)	148.9	156.2	165.4	170.0	172.7	175.6	178

Table 4. South Korea contribution rate in National Health Insurance system, 2009-2015 [13]
[1] The insurance contribution for self-employed is calculated based on the householder's income (property, income, vehicle, age, and gender). A contribution score should be calculated for self-employed.

	Type	Co-payment
Inpatients		20% of total treatment cost (registered cancer patients 5%; registered rare/incurable diseases patients 10%)
Outpatients	Higher level general hospitals	60% of total treatment cost and other expenses
	General hospitals	50% (administrative district: Dong); 45% (administrative district: Eup, Myeon)of total care benefit expenses
	Pharmacy	40% (administrative district: Dong) 35% (administrative district: Eup, Myeon)of total care benefit expenses
	Hospital	30% of total care benefit expenses
	Clinics	30% of total care benefit expenses

Table 5. South Korea *co-payment for inpatients and outpatients [13]
* Co-payment ceiling system: NHI would cover the excess payment in case the patient payment exceeds the government set upper limit

new drugs. Their other duties include healthcare safety research, comparative effectiveness research, economic evaluation, evidence based health policy research, healthcare evidence dissemination research and research collaboration. The collaboration research is conducted with either domestic or international organizations on selected research topics. National Health Insurance System in South Korea as a whole is represented in Figure 1.

Another division is called Division New Health Technology Assessment for systematic review of new medical technology. It refers to health technology assessment, under the Medical Service Act, for new medical services, pharmaceuticals and medical materials. The methodologies used in HTA assessment include systematic literature review, assessment and synthesis of clinical efficacy, critical appraisal of evidence, amalgamation of ethical, organizational, and patient perspectives, and economic evaluation using Korean data. Since June 2010, the task of health technology assessment was transferred from

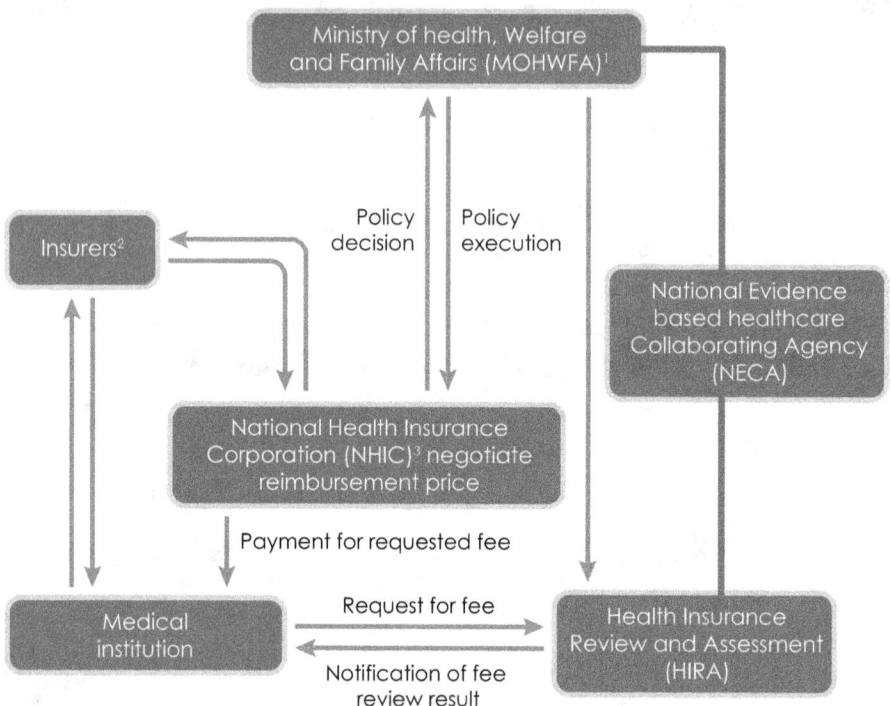

Figure 1. National Health Insurance System in South Korea in 2014
[1] Decision of NHI policies; Approval of insurance rate, criteria for coverage, NHIC budget and regulations; Assessment on new drugs
[2] 3 types of insurance program i.e. Employee Scheme (1977), Social Health Insurance (1981), National Health Insurance (1989)
[3] Review and assess reimbursement price and medical services

HIRA to NECA, which by 2014, has about 100 staff working in the division. HTA process in South Korea is represented in Figure 2.

For the evolution of their healthcare structure, South Korean patients might not feel as much price pressure as their government does in the national insurance system. The government's determination on containing healthcare cost first emerged in the late 1990s. Since the National Health Insurance Act was introduced in 1999, the government has successfully transformed the health insurance system from being managed by multi-insurers to single insurer. It has worked progressively to improve the efficiency of the healthcare services while curbing the rising spending on health insurance. The most noted achievement is probably the cost-savings from its price-cut measures. Drug price in South Korea is one of the lowest in the Asia Pacific region. Effectively, it becomes one of the international reference price countries for Taiwan, Australia, and China, even though

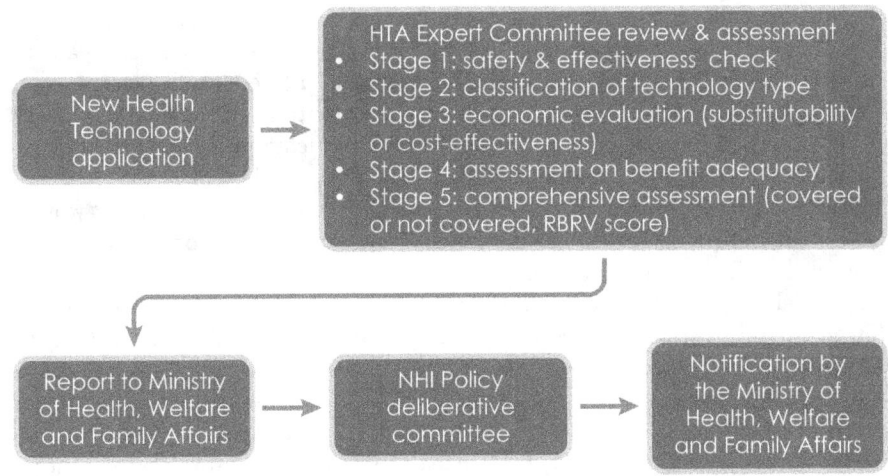

Figure 2. New health technology assessment process (including Resource-Based Relative Value scores) in South Korea

the international reference pricing policy is not officially in place in China. South Korea also takes up a leading role on quality assessment of healthcare benefit. It leverages its experience in health insurance programs in the past 10 years and provide trainings for other developing countries in the region in healthcare performance improvement; such as how to operate and utilize the IT system efficiently for claim reviews, resources, and benefit management, etc.

In this respect, South Korea is exerting an immerse impact on the development of health insurance systems in its neighboring emerging markets.

China

In general, pharmaceutical industry is versatile to the fast changing global market environment. Market access in China is relatively more complex.

In the past 18 years, the Chinese government has been updating a variety of stringent cost control polices on healthcare. Its objectives were to improve the quality of healthcare, as well as tackling the compliance issue in hospital drug procurement and physicians treatment choice. Ultimately, it is hoping to improve the situations of excessive prescriptions, limited patient access as well as controlling the inflating healthcare spending in Level III hospitals, which are the big hospitals.

There was a large scale anti-corruption campaign since 2013. Hospitals and physicians are prohibited to receive any rebates from companies, and restricted from generating profits from patients for additional but unnecessary diagnostic tests and treatment, etc.

Since the first National Prescription Guide was released in 2010, there are hospitals rolling out the policy of One Brand per Molecule in their hospital formulary, e.g. Tianjin. More and more hospital procurements have gone through a central tender organized by their regional government. Global budget for hospitals and zero profit margins on drug dispensing are currently at a testing stage in affluent cities such as Shanghai and Beijing, and provinces like Zhejiang, etc. The draft of new pricing guidelines "Method for the Management of Drug Price" was published in 2010 and it might replace the Government Price Method for Medicines (GPMM) which was released in 2000. If it does, it would put an end of the Independent Pricing Scheme. Off-patent originator products might no longer be able to sell at a premium price.

In parallel to the development aforementioned, there are regular mandated price cuts enforced by National Development & Reform Committee. NDRC is a central government department that formulates the economic and social policies as well as directing the structural reforms in China. Its scope of work also includes monitoring and regulating consumer and drug prices. From 1998 to 2014, NDRC had already conducted almost 32 rounds of drug price cut, which involved over 1,000 drugs under review. Recently, it is targeting on the price of high-cost drugs, such as those for oncology treatment, off-patent original drugs, respiratory treatment, etc. The implementation of these cost-containing measures are carried out by provincial governments. Given the general discrepancies between central government directives and local government execution of those directives that existed, the format and the scale of implementation of the cost cutting measures are subject to the interpretation of the local governments. Consequently, the impact of these cost-containment measures vary across provinces and cities. It places a significant negative effect on the market dynamics of China.

In general though, one could say with some justification that China is progressing towards the direction of rational assessment of drug value. There are several HTA institutes and initiatives set-up, such as WHO Collaborating Center for Health Technology Assessment and Management in Shanghai [14], Shanghai Health Technology Assessment Center, China Evidence-based Medicine Center, Key lab of Health Technology Assessment which is affiliated with the former Ministry of Health, and Pharmacoeconomic Evaluation & Research Center in Fudan University. There are also seven other universities which have their own HTA centers. A number of local governments have set up their local HTA committees, and they include the provinces of Zhejiang, Shaanxi, Liaoning, Shangdong, Jiangsu, Hubei, and the municipal city of Chonqing. A number of *ad hoc* reviews on new medical technology have been carried out, such as the research study on Da Vinci surgical robot in prostate cancer treatment in 2012.

Unfortunately, these HTA efforts are not managed in a coordinated and systematic way. So far, market access in China is not strongly linked to pharmacoeconomic (PE) evaluation of the drug. The international PE data, to some extent, seemed to serve as a reference for the drug application for getting on the positive list of formulary in National Reimbursement Drug List (NRDL). China has seldom used cost-effectiveness concepts such as cost per quality adjusted life year in the national price and reimbursement assessment. In 2012, the National Development & Reform Commission had once asked the pharmaceutical companies to provide the retail (reimbursement) prices of their marketed products in ten countries, which are Canada, France, Germany, Hong Kong, Japan, Korea, Taiwan, U.K., U.S. and the company's country of origin. Although there was no subsequent development since then, there is an expectation within the industry that the central government might consider to implement international reference pricing.

To understand the market access in China, it is important to understand the three different types of health insurance schemes and the two sets of national drug lists.

The three main types of health insurance schemes are Urban Basic Health Insurance Scheme, New Rural Cooperative Medical Scheme, and Urban Residents Basic Medical Insurance. UBHIS and URBMI are for the urbanites, and their coverage extend to 32.36% of total population in 2013. NRCMS is the largest health insurance scheme and mainly provide some forms of health services for the rural population. Its coverage extends to 62.56% of the total population [15]. The two sets of national drug list are taken as the basis for reimbursement formulary. One is the National Essential Drug List, and the other is the National Reimbursement Drug List.

NRDL is the national reimbursement list which comprises all the reimbursed drugs on the three health insurance schemes. The local formulary of these health insurance schemes chooses the reimbursed drugs from NRDL. The decision making criteria for NRDL so far is neither specified nor transparent. The NRDL review process is believed to be through a panel of medical experts and provincial administrators of about 200 people, who are appointed by National Health and Family Planning Commission (i.e. ex-Ministry of Health). Again, one believes that the international PE data were considered. Other plausible factors seem to be drug safety, efficacy, clinical needs, and budget impact analysis. NRDL were updated in 2004 and in 2009. The next version of NRDL had long been anticipated, as it was supposed to be updated again in 2014. As this book goes into print, there is yet no news on the update of the NRDL.

There are two lists of drug in NRDL. List A, according to the latest version of NRDL released in 2009, includes 349 western drugs (positive list) and 154 Traditional Chinese Medicine (TCM) drugs (negative list). They are considered as the basic essential drugs and are fully reimbursed. Most NEDL products are found on List A in NRDL. The drugs on List B are also regarded as essential for medical treatment, but they are mostly high-priced drugs, with a lower reimbursement rate. Patients and their employers or local governments are co-paying the "non-covered" treatments. In 2009, there are 791 western drugs and 833 TCM on List B of NRDL.

Provincial governments could decide the reimbursement rate and adjust the drug price of products on List B (5% price variance) based on NRDL recommended price. Moreover, provincial governments could expand the number of drugs on List B (in principle, it should allow 15% variance compared to drug listing NRDL). In this Provincial Reimbursement Drug List (PRDL), they could determine the price of these newly added drugs on their exclusive local List B. Local governments are entitled with certain degree of autonomy to build a "tailor-made" provincial reimbursement drug list as they see fit for their local market needs.

The last updated NRDL was in 2009. Since then, many drugs are waiting for the opportunity to get access on to the national reimbursement list. It leaves the provincial List B as a viable alternative route for new product launch and get into the reimbursement list in some parts of China. For example, Shanghai is a popular "regional" market chosen by multinational pharmaceutical companies for their new product launch. By 2014, Shanghai has added twice drugs on List B in their local reimbursement list, with about 1,845 molecules; compared with 791 molecules in the NRDL List B in 2009 [16].

For innovative drugs, some companies choose to negotiate a reimbursement status and reimbursement price with the local governments directly. For example, the provincial government of Jiangxi and the city of Qingdao are open to direct negotiations. This method is frequently used on the launch of new oncology drugs. The drug price is agreed upon and then it is translated into a subsidy within the patient assistance program (e.g. Novartis's Glivec, Bayer's Nexavar). This direct negotiation with local government departments (e.g. Provincial Pricing Bureau and Bureau of Human Resources and Social Security) then becomes an alternative pathway of market access, and it is not stated on government guidelines.

Quite easily being confused with NRDL, NEDL refers to the list of essential basic drug that is available and accessible for basic treatments. NEDL is targeting the rural population and low-income patients in Community Health Centers (CHC). Drug price on NEDL is referring to the retail price determined by the government. To keep the drug price low on NEDL, hospitals and CHC are not allowed to mark-up on the retail drug price. NEDL is often the focus for mandatory price-cut by NDRC. The NEDL is updated every three years and the latest update was in 2012 (published in 2013). The coverage of this updated NEDL is closer to what World Health Organization (WHO) suggested as the essential drug list for developing countries. Compared to the last version of NEDL, which was published in 2009, the new list has expanded from 307 molecules to 520 molecules. It listed 317 western drugs, including biologics, and 203 Traditional Chinese Medicines (TCMs). This latest version of the list has for the first time included treatment drugs for cancer, blood disease, end-stage renal disease, and psychiatric disease.

Local governments adapted the newly released NEDL and then published their Provincial Essential Drug Lists (PEDLs) individually. Many provincial governments further expanded the essential drug list by adding more than 100 molecules for their local markets. While most of the provinces have broadened their PEDLs, a few provincial and municipal governments, such as the provinces of Shaanxi and Hunan, and the city of Shanghai, have followed and adapted the complete set of NEDL without making any changes.

To improve the patient access of medical treatment, the central government is promoting the use of NEDL at all levels of hospitals. NHFPC set the purchase target on the new NEDL being 40-50% of all prescribed drugs by volume in Level I & Level II Hospitals, which are county and city level hospitals; and 25-30% of the prescribed drugs in Level III Hospitals, which are the provincial level hospitals and the big hospitals of the region. The effect on actual improvement of patient access is not yet known. But it is projected that the prescription volume on NEDL should increase. This, effectively, would change the market access pathway for multinational pharmaceuticals. The industry seems to be getting more receptive to the idea of bidding under the NEDL tender, putting up a fierce competition with local low-cost drug manufacturers.

The general pathway of market access in China involves government departments both at the central government level and at the provincial and municipal governments levels. The central government departments are responsible for policy formulation and monitoring of policy implementation. The provincial government departments are responsible for implementation and execution of the central government policies in the local market context. This implementation is mainly financed using the local budget.

The health insurance schemes are managed by different government departments. National Health and Family Planning Commission is established in March 2013 from the merger of the Ministry of Health (MOH) and the National Population and Family Planning Commission (NPFPC). It became a new central government agency responsible for healthcare directly reporting to the State Council. It also manages the health insurance for the rural population, which is the NRCMS, compiling the National Essential Drug List and recommending the reimbursed drug price. Among all these healthcare related duties, there is a very important task added to NHFPC. It is to coordinate the health and medical reforms, which was previously a mandate of NDRC.

The monitoring of drug safety duties have been transferred to the China Food and Drug Administration (CFDA), which was formerly known as the State Food and Drug Administration (SFDA) and affiliated to the ex-MOH. Besides the enforcement of current Good Manufacturing Practice (cGMP) requirement to improve the drug quality, they are doing an on-going re-assessment of generic drugs registered in 2007 or after. It is to ensure the marketed products have a bio-equivalence standard with the originator. CFDA is now an independent government agency and seems to be getting more weight as a central government organization. Centre for Drug Evaluation (CDE) is reporting to CFDA. CDE is responsible for reviewing new drug applications. The product testing is conducted by the National Institute of Food and Drug Control.

The registration process in China is notoriously lengthy for imported drugs, which refers to all products manufactured outside China. Even the imported drug has already been launched in other countries for a number of years, it would still be considered as a new product in China. In such case, an additional registration trial is required for the registration process, before any marketing authorization is given. It is hard to estimate the lead time required in the registration. Usually, the product launch date would be adjusted as need be in response to the constantly unexpected hiccups occurred in the review process.

Ministry of Human Resources and Social Security (MOHRSS) is responsible for the management of National Reimbursement Drug List and the health insurance schemes for the urban population, which are UBHIS and URBMI. MOHRSS involves in the decision of UBHIS formulary, which is based on NRDL. They decide the framework for benefits and reimbursement for urban employees and urban residents covered under UBHIS and URBMI.

Regarding the drug price setting process, NDRC is responsible for setting optimal prices for national UBHIS formulary (both List A and B with the exception of Over The Counter—OTC products), drug price for new drugs which are patent protected but are not yet in the local UBHIS formulary. The optimal price is indicative for setting the retail price. There are differences on the drug retail price and manufacturers' selling price, except products on NEDL, which should be maintained as zero mark-up. Since the independent pricing when referring to GPMM is still dependent upon the central government's final approval, patented drugs have the flexibility in setting their drug price if they are proved to have superior efficacy, good quality and safe. The process is that patent drugs should first register their suggested drug price at NDRC before announcing the new drug price in the market.

In practice, the actual drug price setting is highly decentralized. The local drug price is heavily influenced by the Provincial Pricing Bureau and the local provincial government, with restrictions set by the national pricing policies, issued by NDRC. It is estimated that three quarters of the current drug sales are from competitive bidding. Drug price is mostly determined through the bidding process and price negotiation with the stakeholders. The emerging trend is that the central government tends to dedicate the price control to provincial governments from NDRC. In 2014, NDRC already lifted the retail price cap on low-cost drugs. In June 2015, NDRC further announced that they will remove the price control on most of the medicines, but excluding anesthetics and Grade I psychiatric medicines; and will set up a new price monitoring system in the future [17]. The indication is that a new pricing reform on pharmaceutical products is imminent. The pathway of market access in China would undergo further changes.

This is evident from the fact that more and more provincial governments are leading their own negotiations in the local reimbursement drug listing and central tender bidding, the market access to local markets are changing. Some local hospitals have initiated the second round of drug price negotiation for selected products in hospital formulary. Inter-provincial reference pricing has been on trial in a few local markets, e.g. Zhejiang province. All these local cost-containing measures might create further pressure on the drug price, but might shorten the market access process to some local markets eventually. Thus, market access in China is getting diversified but more complicated as a whole. There is no single strategy to access the whole market in the nation. Local governments, such as provincial governments, might even play a more critical role in the market access. They are the crucial gatekeepers for pharmaceutical products listing in the local markets.

In sum, provincial governments decide their own provincial reimbursement drug list, which are drugs on NRCMS formulary and List B on local UBHIS formulary, and that is directly affecting the hospital formulary. They also determine the actual reimbursement rate in List B on the local UBHIS formulary. The provincial governments define the actual drug price by choosing the bidding methods in the provincial level tender; which could be public bidding, bidding by invitations, or direct purchase. The drug prices could also be negotiated directly with the pharmaceutical companies at the provincial level, or the provincial government could directly set the price for OTC drugs on the local UBHIS formulary. Finally, the provincial government has the power to adjust the price on locally added drugs on List B in their UBHIS formulary. Price and reimbursement process in China is summarized in Figure 3.

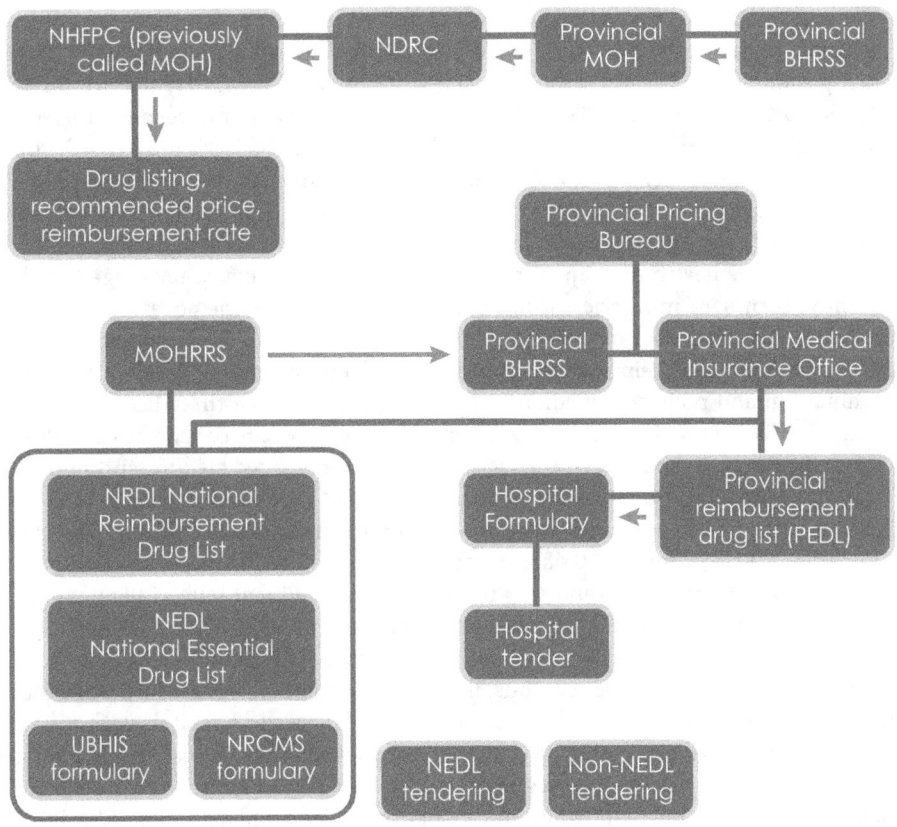

Figure 3. Price and reimbursement process in China

Thailand

The fast development of the health insurance system in Thailand could be an encouraging example for any emerging markets. Since 2002, it has successfully achieved a universal healthcare for about 99% of the total population. The extent of this high healthcare coverage certainly out-performs its neighboring countries which might have a stronger economy and stable political environment. In 2013, the healthcare coverage of the total population in South Korea was 96% and 94.92% in China. [15].

While Thailand compares well with South Korea and China in terms of the extent of its healthcare coverage, its government is under far more financial pressure to maintain its three health insurance schemes. In 2013, the government's share of expenditure on health as a percentage of the total expenditure on health was 80.1%, compared to 55.8% in China and 53.4% in South Korea [4]. Thailand has a fully funded Universal Coverage

Scheme and Civil Servants Medical Benefits Scheme, and it also has a heavily subsidized Social Security Scheme. Given that the healthcare spending is financed by a percentage of the general taxation as well as 2% of tobacco and alcohol consumption tax, the healthcare spending is outpacing its economic growth. For example, the real GDP growth for Thailand was 6.5% in 2012 and 2.9% in 2013, whereas the growth of government spending on healthcare was 9.6% in 2011, an estimated 18% in 2012 and 8.3% in 2013 [4]. The dilemma for the government is how to maintain the patient's access to healthcare services and to improve the healthcare package, while at the same time, contain or even reduce the spiraling healthcare spending.

There are three health insurance schemes in Thailand and they are managed by three different government ministries. It has been the intention for the government to integrate the three health insurance schemes into one single scheme. However, due to the differences in benefits and reimbursement process of all the schemes, it would require great determination and political expediency to achieve the goal. The three health insurance schemes are Civil Servants Medical Benefits Scheme, Social Security Schemes and Universal Coverage Scheme. Apart from the fact that they are managed by different ministries, the amount of resources allocated to support these health schemes also vary.

CSMBS is the health insurance scheme serving civil servants and their families. It covers about 7 million people or 10.45% of total population. It is managed by Comptroller General's Department, direct reporting to the Ministry of Finance. It is fully financed by government taxes. Unlike under CSMBS coverage, patients enrolled either in SSS or in UCS are required prior registration at specific hospitals and are not free to choose the hospital unless it is for emergency. Thus, in terms of flexibility, it is an advantage for patients with the CSMBS scheme who could have direct access to hospitals with the most advanced medical facilities for treatment, which are usually the regional and general hospitals. With CSMBS, it is fee-for-service on outpatients services reimbursement and follows DRG (Diagnosis-Related Group) in inpatients service reimbursement. CSMBS used to spend more on drug purchase than the other two schemes. They included original drugs from multinational pharmaceutical companies in their reimbursement. The price of original drugs was often negotiated and determined individually in CSMBS tenders. However, this scenario is undergoing changes when the government tries to contain the cost on public healthcare spending, and that extends to include drug use in all types of health insurance schemes. Effectively, CSMBS is being targeted for cost control. The government is also cutting down the public spending on all government and teaching hospitals, which directly affects the health benefits under the CSMBS scheme. Hospitals in the public sector should now consider drugs on NLED or generics as their first treatment option. This reduces the level of prescription of original drugs.

At present, Thailand restricts the usage of all medicines in government hospital, with 80% of the drugs should come from NLED. This restriction also applies to teaching hospitals, with 70% of the drugs should come from NLED. The prescription of high-price original drugs is hence significantly reduced. Prior approval is required for using original drug for treatment in some areas, such as hypertension (especially the use of ACE-inhibitors, angiotensin receptor blockers), anti-dyslipidemia treatment (especially the use of statins), anti-inflammation (especially the use of nonsteroidal anti-inflammatory drugs) for arthritis or osteoarthritis, anti-coagulation drugs and anti-cancer drugs, etc.

SSS is the second largest health insurance scheme and covers employees in the private sector. Both employers and employees equally contribute 1.5% of the salary payment, with the maximum salary contribution being 15,000 baht or US$ 444. About 11 million people are insured in SSS. It accounts for 16.42% of the total population and they are mostly young people, who have less demand on health benefits. SSS is managed by the Social Security Office in the Ministry of Labor and Social Welfare. However, the operation of Ministry of Labor and Social Welfare is often disrupted by a change of ruling political party. For that reason, least improvement has been made on health benefits in SSS.

Ministry Of Public Health (MOPH) is responsible for the formulation of healthcare policy, and under it, the National Health Security Office manages UCS, the largest health insurance scheme in the country. It covers the remaining 50 million people or 74.62% of the total population which are not covered by SSS and CSMBS. The funding of UCS is mainly coming from NHSO, partially and occasionally from other government departments or organizations, such as Thai Health Promotion Foundation, National Council for Peace and Order, etc. With 153.2 billion baht or US$ 4.53 billion, the budget for UCS is getting lower in 2015 as it had a planned budget of 183.1 billion baht or US$ 5.42 billion. It had a budget of 154.3 billion baht or US$ 4.56 billion in 2014. The challenge to sustain the same level of service and health benefits in UCS will likely continue.

For the market access into the Thai healthcare market, National List of Essential Drugs is the major channel for getting into the national reimbursement scheme. NLED is listed by INN (International Nonproprietary Name) in therapeutic categories. It is basically a combined drug list, with references to both the suggested essential drugs list from WHO and the recommended list from several local drug committees. The exact process of com-

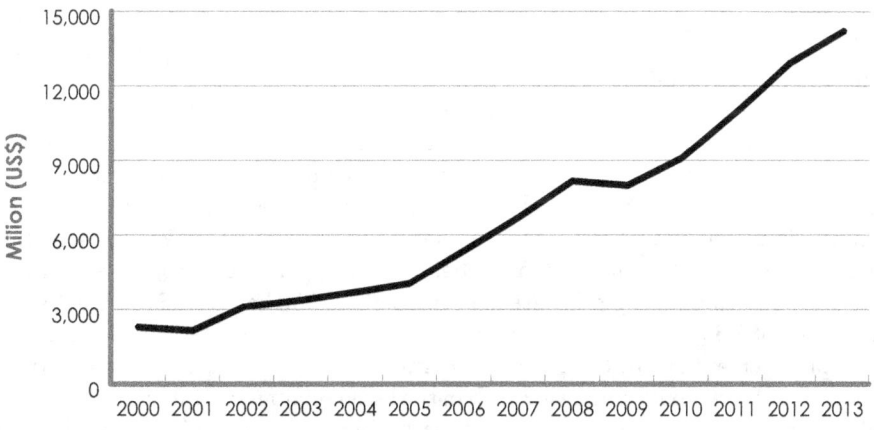

Figure 4. Thailand general government expenditure on health 2000-2013 in current US$ million [4]

piling the drug list is not disclosed. The NLED is in principle reviewed every year, but the last update of NLED was in 2013. The National Drug System Development Committee (NDSDC) was formed in 2012 and it became the first government unit dedicated for the development of NLED. They organize with the expert groups, principally physicians and health economists, with the pharmaceutical industry to assess the drug benefits.

Pharmacoeconomics (PE) data were first used in 2008 in the NLED drug review and assessment process. At that time, only six groups of drugs were requested to submit their PE data, i.e. statins, insulin analogs, hepatitis A and B drugs, osteoporosis treatment, Alzheimer disease treatment and recombinant human erythropoietin. The criteria of assessment were concerning the drug Information, SAFety and ease of use, Efficacy (ISafE) and the Essential Medical Cost Index (EMCI) [18]. Thus, the focus was more on measuring the Quality Adjusted Life Years (QALY) with a cost-effectiveness ceiling, which was 160,000 baht or US$ 4,734.

Since the set-up of the Health Intervention and Technology Assessment Program in 2007, the government has developed a local guideline in 2012 and the latest update was in early 2015. The program is based on the WHO guideline in defining the ICER that should be no more than the GDP *per capita* as a basis of deciding the cost-effective ratio of the drug. It seems the process is progressing to more clarity on the requirements in drug benefits assessment.

Although the Thai government has started drug reviews and assessment processes with considering PE data for almost 7 years, the PE data are not a mandatory requirement for drug application. It is not an indispensable source of information which would affect the decision on NLED. Nevertheless, the pharmaceutical industry is invited to submit PE data with their drug application, but on a voluntary basis. The country is still developing their capacity in Health Technology Assessment (HTA). It is as yet difficult for government institutions to handle the huge demand of drug reviews and assessment with limited patient data and PE expertise in the country. The primary consideration of assessment seems to rely more on budget impact analysis. After the drug is listed on NLED, it is then a guarantee access to all three health insurance schemes. All hospitals formularies include NLED.

Drug price on NLED is the reimbursement price. The price is first calculated based on the median price of the reference countries. Another formula is then applied for re-calculation with reference to the estimated prescription volume. The exact formula used in the calculation process is not publicized. Once this reimbursement price is set, the government hospitals would take this price as a base for negotiation with the manufacturers or use this price as the starting price for tenders. The hospital tenders could be carried out by individual hospitals for a purchase budget from 100,000 baht or US$ 2,959, to 2 million baht or US$ 59,161. Otherwise, they could opt for a national tender, electronic-auction or procurement via the Government Pharmaceutical Organization (GPO). Normally, the final drug price would end up lower than the listed reimbursement price. Pharmaceutical companies could adjust their price upwards, but they are required to apply for approval from the Internal Trade Department beforehand on any price increase. This process is lengthy and requires a very detailed cost structure to support the price increase.

	South Korea	Thailand
New drug application	Registration at Ministry of Food and Drug Safety (MFDS) **Estimated 52-78 weeks (chemicals and biologics)**	Registration at Thai Food and Drug Administration (FDA) **Estimated 64-78 weeks (chemicals) Estimated 104 weeks (biologics)**
Reimbursement drug listing	National Health Insurance (NHI) listing **Estimated 52 weeks**	National List Essential Drugs (NLED) **Estimated 104-156 weeks**
Remarks	Application for NHI listing should be done upon the approval on new drug registration	Application for NLED could be done in parallel with the new drug registration
Estimated total time needed for market access	**Minimum time 104 weeks**	**Minimum time 104 weeks**

Table 6. Estimated timeline from new drug application to gaining access to reimbursement drug listing in South Korea and Thailand

National Data Clearing House is a new concept to support the price and reimbursement review process. It is a new government organization set up officially in 2014 and deals with the budget and financial transactions of the three national health insurance schemes. Ministry Of Public Health (MOPH) plans to establish a National Information Centre and it would be affiliated with the National Clearing House. This is intended to collect patient records and drug use data from the three health insurance schemes. When it is set up, it should resolve the current problems of insufficient patient data in assessing the rational use of drugs. Unfortunately, this new data collection agency has not been approved by the Office of the Public Sector Development Commission (OPSDC) as yet.

For the market access pathway in Thailand, a multi-stakeholders decision making process is often the case. For example, healthcare policy formulation is considered a major duty for MOPH, but the actual decision making process involves several government agencies. This include the Health System Research Institute (HSRI), Thai Health Promotion Foundation, National Health Commission Office (NHCO), and Emergency Medical Institute of Thailand (EMIT). This multi-agency involvement tends to prolong the decision making process in improving the efficiencies. Indirectly, it also delays the harmonization progress of the three national health insurance schemes.

It is also strikingly similar with the case of new drug application. For the first step to access the market in Thailand, pharmaceutical companies are required to submit their application with the (Thailand) Food and Drug Administration (FDA). There are a total 16 sub-committees under FDA [19] responsible for the review and approval of different categories of drugs, such as modern medicines, traditional Thai medicines and herbal med-

	South Korea	China	Thailand
New drug application	Korea Food and Drug Administration (KFDA)	China Food and Drug Administration (CFDA)	Food and Drug Administration (FDA) Thailand
Formulation of health insurance and reimbursement policy	Ministry of Health, Welfare and Family Affaires (MOHWFA)	National Health and Family Planning Commission (NHFPC) and National Development and Reform Commission (NDRC)	Ministry Of Public Health (MOPH), Health System Reform Office (HSRO), Emerging Medical Institute of Thailand (EMIT), National Health Commission Office (NHCO) and Thai Health Promotion Foundation
Management of health insurance	National Health Insurance Corporations (NHIC)	NHFPC and Ministry Of Human Resources and Social Security (MOHRSS) provides framework of health insurance schemes[1]	Comptroller General's Office, Social Security Office (SSO), National Health Security Office (NHSO), National Data Clearing House
Reimbursement drug listing review and assessment	Health Insurance Review and Assessment Service (HIRA) and National Evidence based healthcare Collaborating Agency (NECA)	NHFPC provides guidance, implementation by Provincial governments, Provincial BHRSS and Provincial Bureau Health and Family Planning Commission (BHFPC)	National Drug System Development Committee (NDSDC), Committee of National Experts
Reimbursement price setting	Mainly led by NHIC[2]	Pricing guidance given by NDRC[3]	Subcommittee of National List of Essential Drugs (NLED)[4]

Table 7. Structure of decision making in market access

[1] Implementation by Provincial Bureau Human Resources and Social Security (BHRSS) and Provincial Medical Insurance Bureau

[2] Pricing decision would be affected by the recommendations from HIRA

[3] Final pricing decision would be subject to Provincial Pricing Bureau, Provincial Finance Bureau, Provincial BHRSS, Provincial BHFPC, and local hospitals procurement would further negotiate drug price

[4] Pricing decision would be affected by the recommendations from Health Intervention and Technology Assessment Program (HITAP)

icines, and so on. Including the two-year safety monitoring period, a new drug approval for registration might possibly take two to four years, plus further two years in getting listed in NLED. Besides the stringent drug cost containment measures, the lengthy process is another critical factor for consideration of market access in Thailand.

Table 6 compares the timing from new drug application to gaining access to reimbursement drug listing in South Korea and Thailand.

A further comparison, including also China, is made in Table 7 about the structure of decision making in market access.

Challenges and catalyzers for Market Access

Given the increasingly affluent economies in some Asian emerging markets, multinational pharmaceutical companies might not anticipate the degree of austere atmosphere in healthcare would be as much as they have to face in the other developed markets in Europe. In fact, the challenges for market access might not be less in the Asian emerging markets, although quite possibly, the nature of these challenges is different from other market regions.

If one says the access to Asian markets is moving towards an evidence-based assessment on health benefits, the primary challenge would be how to build up the local capacity in this new knowledge area, including having both local PE experts and PE data available for the pharmaceutical companies and the health insurance review agencies. The degree to which a country has attained this goal would be a good indicator if the country is ready to implement a rational reimbursement review and assessment with the use of PE data. Compared with the U.K. (NICE was set up in 1999), Asia is about 10 years late in developing evidence-based assessment, although governments in Asia have already raised their awareness of using economic assessment on drug spending.

A good example is South Korea: its government has actively initiated a regional network with Taiwan and Japan for the regular exchange of HTA studies. This is to acknowledge the problems of limited national PE data, hence borrowing the experience from their neighboring countries which have similar healthcare structures and comparable socio-economic background.

This solution might not be applicable to some low to middle income countries, like Thailand. HTA data from East Asia might not be fully transferrable to the South East Asia, and its neighboring countries have yet to initiate enough HTA studies. One major challenge for Thailand is the lack of PE experts and a nationwide database of PE data. Most of the local PE studies are focused on the affluent cities, which do not reflect the medical needs of the entire country. Due to concerns on private data protection, Thai patient data is used to be restricted for pharmaceutical companies. Without the access of patient outcome data, it is rather difficult to make any treatment comparisons possible. The government has planned to set up a National Information Centre. If so, it could collect patient outcome data systematically and drug usage data from prescription tracking.

Certainly, it would take time for the quality of data to improve. For users of healthcare statistics, it is imperative that they should understand how the data is collected in order to determine their margin of error. The credibility of PE data in Thailand and China is the lacking of relevant market data that could be validated. In the 1980s, the Chinese Central Government has dedicated a certain degree of autonomy to the local government administration in their social, economic and healthcare development [20]. Within each level of the local government, there is a statistics bureau for data collection of the region and data analysis. These data would then pass onto the statistics bureau at the next administrative level, and eventually to the National Bureau of Statistics and other government ministries. This structure gives rise to a contradictory role for the local bureaux. On the one hand, the data it generates facilitate a better understanding by the Central Government on the local region. On the other hand, the Central Government also uses the same data to assess the performance of the local government, on their level of achievement concerning the social and economic objectives set by the Central Government every year. Given that the local bureaux are mainly staffed by people from the area, and also that failing to attain the target given is likely to draw criticisms from the Central and the local government, the local bureaux would tend to align their interests with those of the local government. This resulted in data inflation, or data deflation, that is so often found in Chinese statistics.

Another challenge for market access in China is the absence of a systematic national drug price database. It is difficult to make any inference for the drug price set in different cities and to understand the local drug price development. In most cases, the pharmaceutical companies would need to spend extra resources to collect and to manage the pricing data themselves.

Pharmaceutical companies might hesitate to spend more resources on collecting data for PE studies if the PE data is not a mandatory requirement for new drug applications. It might not justify in conducting pharmacoeconomic studies either if the pharmaceutical market size is too modest. Without the collaborative efforts from the pharmaceutical industry, this would be difficult for some emerging markets in Asia like Thailand, Indonesia, and Vietnam to have a major breakthrough on HTA. It is expected that market access would still heavily rely on budget impact analysis and direct price negotiation in most emerging markets in Asia.

Along with the use of evidence based assessment on health benefits in 2006, South Korea has built up an advanced IT system to support the tracking of prescription behavior and the collection of drug usage data. It effectively improves the quality of healthcare by reducing the possibilities of inappropriate use of drugs. More importantly, it has reduced the number of over-prescriptions and cut back unnecessary healthcare spending. The South Korean healthcare system is profiting from a sound technology infrastructure, and turns it to a proven efficient system on health benefit assessment and review. It means that a good IT system could be a solution to speed up the process from new drug applications to health benefits reviews and assessments in other Asian markets.

Market access would then be a simpler process for pharmaceutical companies.

Unfortunately, an advanced IT system itself might not solve the problem of lengthy process on new drug applications and applications for reimbursement status in Thailand

and China. In 2014, due to the shortage of drug review experts at CDE in China, there were no approvals given to any new drug applications from multinational pharmaceutical companies.

Their challenges are not just the lacking of an IT infrastructure and experts to support the growing demand on new drug application. They also lack a set of transparent and consistent regulations and guidelines for the industry to follow in price and reimbursement review process. The price setting method on products in NLED in Thailand is an example. The drug price for NLED, in principle, is calculated based on the median price of reference products. However, it could be subject to adjustment (mostly downwards) if there is a generic product in NLED. The responsible authorities do not communicate with the pharmaceutical companies on how and what reference products are actually used in their decisions.

Facing with the fast-changing market environment, not only the pharmaceutical companies but also the Asian governments need to find ways to adapt. This is certainly going to be a long-term process. The Asian governments sometimes need to be very cautious when transferring the market experience and knowledge gained in the western countries. Thailand has introduced the first version of the HTA guide in 2008 and the revised version in 2013, focusing on PE revision. On the latest published HITAP's guideline, it has set the incremental cost-effectiveness ceiling threshold as what WHO suggested, which is no more than the GDP per capita. However, this might not be a practical solution for a lower middle income country. The GDP per capita was US$ 5,779 in Thailand in 2013. This compared with South Korea which has a GDP per capita of US$ 25,977 in the same year. The HITAP's guideline then set the incremental cost-effectiveness ceiling at baht 160,000 or US$ 4,733, which seems to be incongruent with the general economic standard of Thailand.

This reflects that certain level of financial adjustments should be made to bridge the gap in economic assessment on drug value in some emerging markets in Asia. Innovative drugs, like oncology treatment, could only justify its cost using QALY than just looking at the cost effectiveness threshold. In Thailand, the drug price for new treatments would often be perceived as too high and the government would eventually resolve the issue by price negotiation. Economic evaluations tend to over-rule clinical benefits in the assessment process. In order to have a fairer review, evidence based assessment should also be used for price negotiation. A sensible adjustment on the PE guideline would be instrumental for the development of HTA for emerging markets in Asia.

At present, the major challenges for market access in China are the complex tendering systems. There is not a uniform universal process of tendering across the 22 provinces, 4 municipal cities, and 5 autonomous regions (excluding Hong Kong and Macau). The local tenders are implemented in different timeline with different requirements. Pharmaceutical companies have to allocate additional manpower for the tenders in the local regions. This leads to the development of the strategy from pharmaceutical companies of shifting their resources to the most affluent and high potential regions. Unsurprisingly, high quality and advanced treatments are still mostly limited in big cities. Issues of geographical disparity on healthcare service are evident. This would work against the Chi-

	South Korea		China		Thailand	
	Private %	Public %	Private %	Public %	Private %	Public %
2005	47.0	53.0	61.2	38.8	35.6	64.4
2006	45.3	54.7	59.3	40.7	27.3	72.7
2007	45.3	54.7	53.1	46.9	23.7	76.3
2008	45.5	54.5	50.1	49.9	24.1	75.9
2009	43.5	56.5	47.5	52.5	25.8	74.2
2010	43.4	56.6	45.7	54.3	25.4	74.6
2011	44.5	55.5	44.1	55.9	22.3	77.7
2012	45.5	54.5	44.0	56.0	20.5	79.5
2013	46.6	53.4	44.2	55.8	19.9	80.1

Table 8. Private and Government expenditure on health as percentage of total expenditure on health in selected Asian emerging markets 2005-2013 [4]

nese government's wish to improve the healthcare provision across the nation. Providing support for the pharmaceutical companies in market access in remote areas would accelerate the healthcare development in China. There should be a systematic and organized tendering schedule and methods. Information on local tenders should be made available to the industry.

The current priority of the Chinese government is to focus on moving to a market based price setting system instead of the top-down price control. The government believes that it is an effective catalyst for the future market growth. The recent announcement from NDRC on removing price control on most medicine is an encouraging signal for market access. Another catalyst for market access for the country is the government initiative to open up more channels. Chinese government has started to explore additional distribution channels. In mid 2014, there was a draft regulation by CFDA for discussing the possibility of selling prescription drugs via online pharmacy. While one still needs to evaluate this option, the thinking certainly provides a fresh perspective for rural patient access in the vast geographical landscape of China.

Table 8 compares private and government expenditure on health as percentage of total expenditure on health in South Korea, China, and Thailand.

2.5 Market Outlook

The recent trend in emerging markets in Asia is to expand the reimbursement drug list and to extend the reimbursement coverage to different segments of the population.

Governments in Asia are playing a growing significant role of healthcare service. There remains the delicate balance of how to striking a balance between keeping the healthcare spending on check and not lowering the healthcare service quality.

South Korea has successfully contained the pharmaceutical spending and reduced excessive prescriptions in the past decade. But, to a certain extent, the lowering of drug price has made the market somewhat less attractive for the launch of new innovative products. This is reflected in the relative fewer number of new oncology drugs have been launched in South Korea. For the near future, it would be a challenge for the government to develop a win-win strategy which could attain their goals in healthcare development as well as supporting the commercial interest of the pharmaceutical industry.

The trend for drug price is likely to go down across the emerging markets in Asia. This would be driven by market forces instead of austerity measures. Hospitals in South Korea, Thailand and China would become more cost conscious on their budget spending, considering the possibility that practice of global budget might be used in the future. Pharmaceutical industry might well consider different methods to increase their market reach. Both Thailand and China are getting more receptive to patient assistance programs. This would minimize over-relying on price cut. In Thailand, some pharmaceutical companies have introduced special programs in hospitals which ensure the doctors could access their drugs by making them available in the hospital inventory anyway. In China, there are some oncology products selling in the out-of-pocket market, but these products are generally supported by a customized patient assistance program. Pharmaceutical companies provide free medications after the patients completed, and complied with, the basic treatment course.

There is a possibility of implementing reference pricing in China. The implementation is probably in a format of regional reference pricing rather than international reference pricing. The price is likely to compare with other Chinese regions rather than a cross-country reference. Other emerging markets in Asia might also implement some type of price reference but it is likely that they would be limited to references within the Asian region. The most often selected countries in the region for reference are Taiwan and South Korea. They are the two countries with the lowest-drug price in Asia. This could be a potential constraint for the pharmaceutical industry in setting drug price.

Yet, as a whole, the future outlook for emerging markets in the Asian region is optimistic. Their governments are adapting to the changing healthcare environment reasonably fast. The regulatory environment seems to become more transparent and efficient as well. Although the trend for the drug price might seem to go lower, the prescription volume is likely to increase as governments favor increasing healthcare coverage. It would then be a commercial decision for the pharmaceutical industry to define the potential market size, what market segments would be suitable for their products; and strategies like what types of product would be favorable for a low drug price but high sales volume reimbursement market, and what types of product would be better launched in a niche private market at high drug price. All in all, it is anticipated that there should be new types of patient assistance programs evolving that facilitate effective market access.

2.6 References

1. International Financial Corporation. http://www.ifc.org/wps/wcm/connect/corp_ext_content/ifc_external_corporate_site/home (last accessed October 2015)
2. Health outcomes and cost: A 166-country comparison. The Economist, Intelligence Unit. Available at http://www.eiu.com/public/topical_report.aspx?campaignid=Healthoutcome2014 (last accessed October 2015)
3. The World Bank. http://www.worldbank.org (last accessed October 2015)
4. World Health Organization Health Accounts. http://www.who.int/health-accounts/en/ (last accessed October 2015)
5. Central Intelligence Agency, The World Factbook. https://www.cia.gov/library/publications/the-world-factbook/ (last accessed October 2015)
6. China Statistical Year Book 2013. http://www.stats.gov.cn/tjsj/ndsj/2013/indexeh.htm (last accessed October 2015)
7. World Health Organization. Global Health Observatory (GHO) data. Country statistics . http://www.who.int/gho/countries/en/ (last accessed October 2015)
8. Thailand Social Security Office. http://www.sso.go.th/wpr/eng/index.html (last accessed October 2015)
9. Asian Development Bank. Key Indicators for Asia and the Pacific 2014. http://www.adb.org/publications/key-indicators-asia-and-pacific-2014 (last accessed October 2015)
10. Han S, Park J. Government Says "Price of drugs should be reduced if they have low efficacy", While Pharmaceutical companies say "Government decision ignores reality". Donga Ilbo, August 28, 2008. Available at http://members.krpia.or.kr/commons/pop_print.asp?bd_num=1210&bd_id=10 (last accessed October 2015)
11. IMS Market Prognosis 2015-2019 - South Korea. http://www.dailypharm.com/News/198237 (last accessed October 2015)
12. Korean Research-based Pharmaceutical Industry Association (KRPIA). http://www.krpia.co.kr/ (last accessed October 2015)
13. National Health Insurance Service, South Korea. http://www.nhic.or.kr/static/html/wbd/g/a/wbdga0101.html (last accessed October 2015)
14. World Health Organization. Collaborating centres. WHO collaborating centres database. http://www.who.int/collaboratingcentres/database/en/ (last accessed October 2015)
15. Zhao K. HTA experience and impact on health delivery system in China. China Health Technology Assessment Center, National Health Development Research Center, MOH China. July 1, 2013. Available at http://www.gai.nus.edu.sg/niha/wp-content/uploads/2013/07/Prof_ZHAO_Kun.pdf (last accessed October 2015)
16. Lu P. China Pricing and Reimbursement. Datamonitor Healthcare, October 9, 2013. Available at https://service.datamonitorhealthcare.com/geography/china/market-access/pricing-and-reimbursement/ (last accessed October 2015)

17. Dennis M. China to remove price control on most medicines from June 1. First Word Pharma Plus, May 5, 2015. Available at http://www.firstwordpharma.com/node/1267334#axzz3oMJQVVQo (last accessed October 2015)
18. Wibulpolprasert S. The need for guidelines and the use of economic evidence in decision making in Thailand: lessons learnt from the development of the National List of Essential Drugs. *J Med Assoc Thai*, 2008; 91 Suppl 2: S1-S3
19. Food and Drug Administration Thailand. http://www.fda.moph.go.th/eng/index.stm (last accessed October 2015)
20. The development of medical device regulations increase the capability in market supervision (author's translation), China Pharmaceutical News, 8th January, 2009. Available at http://www.zgbzad.com/zgyybw/ (last accessed October 2015)

7 To know more

- Blumenthal D, Hsiao W. Privatization and its discontents--the evolving Chinese health care system. N *Engl J Med* 2005; 353: 1165-70
- Eggleston K. Health Care for 1.3 Billion: An overview of China's Health System. The Walter H Shorenstein Asia-Pacific Research Center, Stanford University, Asia Health Policy Program. Working paper series on health and demographic change in the Asia-Pacific. Asia Health Policy Program working paper #28, January 9, 2012. Available at http://iis-db.stanford.edu/pubs/23668/AHPPwp_28.pdf (last accessed October 2015)
- Health Insurance Review and Assessment service, South Korea. https://www.hira.or.kr/eng/#&panel1-1 (last accessed October 2015)
- Health Intervention and Technology Assessment Program, Thailand. http://www.hitap.net/en/ (last accessed October 2015)
- IMS Market Prognosis 2015-2019 - China, 2015
- IMS Market Prognosis 2015-2019 - Thailand, 2015
- Ministry of Finance website, Thailand. http://www2.mof.go.th/ (last accessed October 2015)
- NHSO Annual Report Fiscal Year 2013. National Health Security Office, Thailand, August 2014. Available at http://www.nhso.go.th/eng/Files/content/255804/7beb65df-fd3e-4871-b7af-9781896ee255-130740737044951250.pdf (last accessed October 2015)
- National Evidence based healthcare Collaborating Agency, South Korea. http://www.inahta.org/our-members/members/neca/ (last accessed October 2015)
- National Health and Family Planning Commission, China. http://en.nhfpc.gov.cn/ (last accessed October 2015)
- National Health Security Office, Thailand. http://www.nhso.go.th/FrontEnd/Default.aspx (last accessed October 2015)
- Ngorsuraches S, Meng W, Kim BY. Drug reimbursement decision making in Thailand, China, and South Korea. *Value Health* 2012; 15(1 Suppl): S120-S125

- South Korea's Economy: What do you do when you reach the top? *The Economist*, Nov 12th, 2011, print edition. Available at http://www.economist.com/node/21538104 (last accessed October 2015)
- Wagstaff A, Bilger M, Buisman L, et al. Who benefits from government health spending and why? A global assessment. Policy Research Working Paper 7044, World Bank Group Development Research Group September 2014. Available at http://elibrary.worldbank.org/doi/abs/10.1596/1813-9450-7044 (last accessed October 2015)
- Xu C. Chinese reform and Chinese regional decentralization. London School of Economics, November 29, 2006. Available at http://policydialogue.org/files/events/Xu_Chinese_Reform_and_Chinese_Regional_Decentralization.pdf (last accessed October 2015)

Market Access in South American Countries

Arturo Schweiger, Alejandro Sonis
With the collaboration of Andrea Induni and Diego Miranda

3.1 Introduction

The present chapter will describe the Health Systems of the South American Countries and their main Economic characteristics related with Macroeconomic Variables, Social Protection and Public and Private Financing Systems. In a second stage, the chapter will focus on Pharmaceutical Markets of selected South American countries.

The South American Countries are included in the Governmental Organization defined as UNASUR. This Organization started on the 17th of December of 2004, in the "III Cumbre Suramericana" in Cuzco (Peru), where the presidents of 12 South American Countries decided to create the Community of the South American Nations. In a second meeting, the Countries met in an Assembly at Isla Margarita (Venezuela) the 17th of April of 2007, reshaped the Community and renamed as the "Union of South American Nations" (UNASUR), based on 12 countries with common languages (Spanish, Portuguese or English). The UNASUR reached a status of observational member at the United Nations (UN) General Assembly, after the area of judicial affairs of UN approved its request.

3.2 General economic outlook

The South American Countries have a territory of 17,738,687 km^2 and a population of 397,529,000 inhabitants. On the Economic dimensions, the UNASUR countries have a GDP of 4,300,000 Billions of dollars. The region of Southern American Countries and the Caribbean Countries is defined as the "Latin American Region" and it was in known in the literature of Health Policies as one of the most inequitable in the world. Even though, over the last decade, the countries of Latin America have made huge advances in reducing poverty and improving social outcomes. The Extreme Poverty fell by more than a third from 19.3% in 2002 to 12.0% in 2014; and the Inequality, as measured by the Gini coefficient, fell from 0.560 to 0.507 in 2010.

The average GDP growth rate for all countries of South America was around 3.8% per year (Figure 1): five countries (Argentina, Bolivia, Brazil, Chile and Colombia) presented an average GDP growth rate per year similar to 3.8% per year for all countries; two countries (Ecuador and Peru) had an average GDP growth rate per year greater than the average GDP growth rate of all 10 countries and the average GDP growth rate per year for three countries (Paraguay, Uruguay and Venezuela); it increased over the period less than the average GDP growth rate for all countries. Moreover, as shown in Figure 1, the dispersion of the average GDP growth rate is very low (the exception is Peru). This average of GDP is high if we compared against the average of North American Free Trade Agreement (NAFTA) and Economic and Monetary Union (EMU), from 2000 to 2010, they were, respectively, 1.9% per year and 1.4% per year.

Rank	Countries	GDP (Bln.$)	Share (%)
1	Brazil	2,243.9	52.18
2	Argentina	611.7	14.22
3	Colombia	378.1	8.79
4	Venezuela	371.3	8.63
5	Chile	277	6.44
6	Peru	200.3	4.66
7	Ecuador	94.5	2.20
8	Uruguay	55.7	1.30
9	Bolivia	30.6	0.71
10	Paraguay	29.2	0.68
11	Suriname	5.3	0.12
12	Guyana	3.1	0.07
Total South America Countries		**4,300.7**	**100.00**

Table 1. Gross Domestic Product (GDP) of South American Countries (source: UNASUR data 2014)

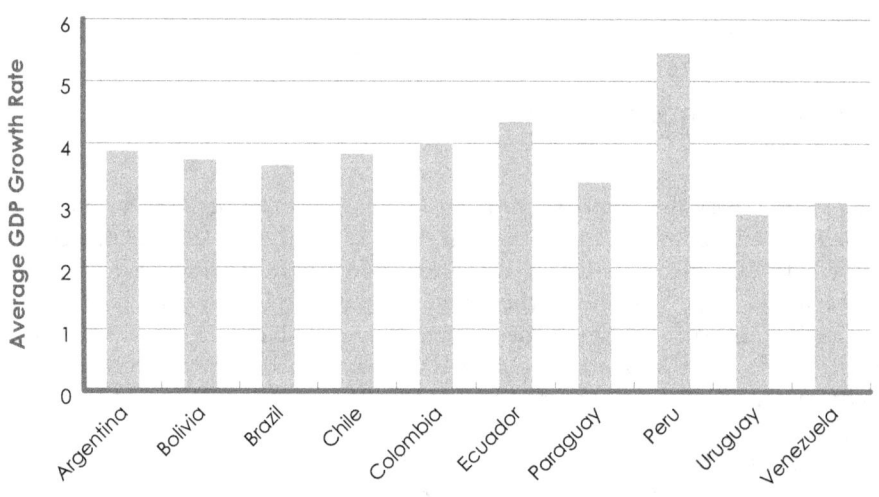

Figure 1. Average Growth Rate. Years 2000-2010

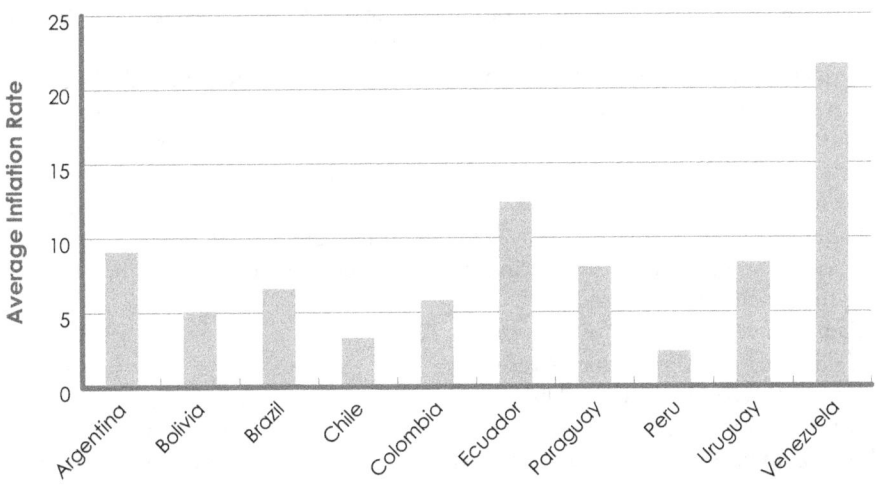

Figure 2. Average Inflation Rate. Years 2000-2010

The average inflation rate for all countries of UNASUR was 8.1% per year, relatively low considering the historically high inflation rates in South America during the 1980s and 1990s; and six countries (Bolivia, Brazil, Colombia, Chile, Peru and Paraguay) had an average inflation rate per year lower than the average inflation of all countries. Two countries (Argentina and Uruguay) had an average inflation rate slightly above the average inflation rate of 8.1% per year; and two other countries, Ecuador and Venezuela, had an average inflation rate per year greater than the average inflation rate of UNASUR countries (12.3% per year and 21.7% per year, respectively). Besides, and as shown in Figure 2, the dispersion of the average inflation rate is relatively low (the exception are Peru and Venezuela).

The unemployment rate was relatively high at the beginning of the 2000s, reaching double digits, for almost all UNASUR countries (the exceptions were Brazil and Paraguay). At the end of the 2000s the unemployment rate for almost all countries, with the exception of Colombia, dropped to figures around a 7.4% per year (average rate).

At the beginning of the 2000s, all UNASUR countries had high current account deficits to GDP. In our view, at least three reasons explain this performance: first, the Argentinean and Brazilian exchange rate crises, respectively in 2001-02 and 2002, ended up affecting the economic dynamics of other countries in the region; second, the slowdown of the world economy, particularly the United States, reduced the demand for South American products; and third the commodity prices (agricultural and mineral – especially copper and iron) of the UNASUR exports fell, basically from 2001 to 2003. In 2005 the current account deficits were reduced and in 2006 and 2007 the current accounts of almost all UNASUR countries (the exceptions were Colombia and Uruguay) turned positive. During this period, the world economy showed high growth and the commodity prices increased considerably. From 2008 to 2010, the current account deteriorated due to the "great recession". Despite this deterioration, the current account deficits were still better than those observed in the beginning of the 2000s.

To conclude this section, it is important to mention that at the end of the 2000s, a set of factors contributed to the convergence of the macroeconomic performance and to face the contagious concerns of the international financial crisis in the main South America countries:

- Lower interest rates;
- Public accounts in general improved with low level of indebtedness;
- Inflation stopped rising (Argentina and Venezuela were the exception); current account deficits were reduced;
- Competitive exchange rates emerged;
- High level of foreign exchange reserves;
- Reduced short-term external liabilities;
- Capital account regulations in place.

The Region of South America benefitted from record world commodity prices thanks to China's ever-growing purchases of oil, soybeans and other raw materials, but now the countries from this region present uncertainty due to the fall of the price of the commodities and the slowdown of the world economy. In China, the slowdown of the Economy continues and there are more downside risks than the market expects for the second half. The U.S. Economy continues to recover and the probability of facing a stronger dollar has increased.

The countries in the Region consider that this Economic Scenario will keep similar conditions in the medium term (next three years), developing an important challenge for the countries in South America to keep pace with their economic growth rate.

3.3 Health Sector

The South American Countries, even if they came from a similar Spanish or Portuguese origin present Health Systems with important differences. The review of the Health Systems will include Argentina, Brazil, Colombia and Venezuela based on their huge impact in the pharmaceutical market, due to the fact that these countries contributed in year 2014 with more than 60% the of the sales of the pharmaceutical industries in Latin America.

The main variables that will be considered in order to describe the health system will be:
- Social Health Protection Systems;
- Types of Social Health Coverage;
- Funding of Health Systems;
- Per Capita Health Funding and Outcomes;
- Private and Government expenditure on health as percentage of total expenditure on Health.

Country	Social health protection – Health coverage
Argentina	**Social Security Subsector:** for workers in the formal market, covers 55% of the population = 12% Provincial Medical Insurance + 34% National Medical Insurance + 9% a health care program for pensioners called PAMI. **Public Subsector:** covers 35% of the population does not have social health insurance, generally those with lower income, although formally universal coverage is considered; extra 2% are covered by government health plans with explicit guarantees: Programa Sumar - Programa Federal de Salud (PROFE). **Private Subsector:** prepaid medicine companies = 8% of the population. National Medical Insurance and prepaid medicine companies must offer the "Programa Médico Obligatorio" (PMO), which establishes medical services bundled.
Brazil	The Sistema Único de Sâude (SUS) has universal coverage with comprehensive care (basic care to highly complex, as organ transplants). With the Citizen Constitution of 1988, which sets health as a universal right and duty of the State, were unified the health institutions of Social Security and the Ministry of Health. In addition to access to SUS, 25% of the population has double coverage, as they buy private individual health insurance or collective (partially with premiums paid by employers).
Colombia	Members of the Sistema General de Seguridad Social en Salud in 2011: 96% of the total population. **Tax regime:** covers 42.6%, for formal sector workers and their families or people with ability to pay. Financed based on corporate contributions and workers. **Subsidized regime:** covers 48.4%, to cover the poor and vulnerable with no ability to pay. **Special regimes:** they cover 4.8%, including independent health systems forces military, teachers and employees of the Colombian oil company. Since 2007 -coverage insurance partial extension funded by federal subsidies. The Plan Obligatorio de Salud (POS), subsidized regime, corresponds to 60% of the POS tax regime. For 2012, the capitation payment unit had an average value of USD 266 for the tax system and $ 159 for subsidized.
Venezuela, BR	The National Health Plan assumes the strategy "Barrio Adentro" to build new institutional health and linchpin of the Sistema Público Nacional de Salud (SPNS), with a model of comprehensive and continuous care, with emphasis on comprehensive outpatient quality care, family and community, with free universal coverage. Instituto Venezolano de los Seguros Sociales (IVSS), an autonomous body under the Ministry People's Power for Labor, was created to provide health services to formal workers at the national level, whether public or private, and their families, however, by decision of Government, since 2000 the agency provides health services to the entire population that requires it. In the SPNS services are organized through a network stratified by level of complexity where all service providers are articulated under the principles of reciprocity, complementarities, solidarity and equity. In addition to universal coverage SNPS, estimates for 2005 indicated that 32% of the population had some form of health insurance: IVSS covered 17.5% of the population, private health insurance to 11.7% and 2.4% of the population had double coverage (IVSS and private insurance). Instituto de Previsión y Asistencia Social del Ministerio de Educación and Instituto de Previsión Social de las Fuerzas Armadas are descentralice management bodies attached to Ministerio del Poder Popular para la Educación y para la Defensa, respectively, providing health services to the population affiliated and their families.

Table 2. Social Health Protection Systems in Southern American Countries

Country	Coverage by social insurance (welfare or social security)	Insurance coverage focused on poverty population or specific group	Ministry of health coverage and subnational government levels	Coverage by private and prepaid insurance
Argentina	55% Social Insurances	2% with explicit guarantees: Programa Sumar - Programa Federal de Salud (PROFE)	Universal Access (mostly 35% without any other coverage)	8%
Brazil	-	-	100% SUS universal Access (mainly 75% without any other coverage)	25% (paid by companies or individuals volunteer)
Colombia	42,6 %tax regime (public or private insurance) 4% special regime	48,4% subsidized regime (funded with fiscal resources, cross-subsidies and contributions)	-	3% private volunteer insurance
Venezuela, BR	30% IVSS, IPASME, IPSFA	-	SPNS universal coverage, integrated IVSS services	Private insurance, insurance premiums canceled by private or public companies or state bodies.

Table 3. Types of Social Health Coverage in Southern American Countries

In Table 2 the Social Health Protection Systems are described for the selected countries. From the information presented, in all the four countries the Government has an important role in the Health Insurance Services, in the delivery of Health Services and in the purchase of drugs and treatments from the pharmaceutical industries.

In the Table 3 the Social Health Coverage indicates that Brazil is the country that has developed a system with the largest participation of the Government Funding and that the other three countries share mix systems with multiple source of coverage.

The Table 4 explains the characteristics of the funding of the health Protection in the different countries, including some details about the copayments in each countries.

In Table 5 some additional Economics and Performance indicators are presented related with the measures of per capita expenditure and the level of these countries in terms of spending rank and of health outcomes rank developed by the literature.

The information provided by Table 6 verifies the evolution of the total health expenditure that has to be financed by the private sector in the four main pharmaceutical markets during the period 2005 to 2014. The review of the table shows that there is a reduction in the indicator of the expenditure in health financed by the private sector in the

Country	Funding: participation in GDP, health expenditure composition and sources
Argentina	**Total expenditure on health:** according to several estimates, the total expenditure on health services in Argentina, measured as a percentage of GDP for 2009 is between 8.6% and 9.4%. **Public spending on health**, added to social security, has average share of order of 4.8% of GDP, standing out 2009 as the year of greater participation with 6.2%. In 2003 and 2004 recorded the slightest relevance to 4.3% and 4.2%, respectively. **Public spending on health,** including social security, accounts for approximately 70%of total health spending. **Private expenditure on health:** between 35% and 28% of pocket expense. **Sources:** Public Health Care: general revenue and international credits. National social insurance: worker contributions (3% of salary) and employer (6% of salary). PAMI-INSSJP: contributions of active workers (5% of salary, 3% and 2% personal contribution employer);the contribution of pensioners, which vary between 6% and 3% of their income; and contributions of national treasure. **Free** public services.
Brazil	**Total health expenditure** as a proportion of GDP in 2008 was 8.4%. Public health funding is 3.67% of GDP, with the participation of the Federal Government (1.67%), States (0.93%) and Municipalities (1.07%).This corresponds to 56% of private expenditure and 44% public expenditure on health. **Sources:** The SUS is financed by the three spheres of government: the Union covers 44.8% of expenditure with actions and health services, States 25.6% and Municipalities 29.6% (2008). Federal funding sources are social taxes, such as the Contribution tax payments for Social Security Financing (Cofins) (35%), Contribution on net income of companies (CSLL) (35%) and tax sources (20%). **Free** public services.
Colombia	**Total expenditure on health** is between 7% (2010) and 6.4% of GDP (2009). **Public expenditure** corresponds to 84% of total health expenditure and private expenditure to 16% of total health expenditure (2009). **Sources:** tax regime - contributions from employers (8.5%) and employees (4%) on the monthly salary, pensioners trading at 12% of income; subsidized system – resources national tax transferred to departments and municipalities, own resources subnational areas and 1.5 points of the contribution of members of the contributory regime, that are transferred to the subaccount of Solidarity FOSYGA (Fondo de Seguridad y Garantía en Salud) to contribute to the funding of beneficiaries of the subsidized regime. **There are co-payments.**
Venezuela, BR[1]	Public funding of social programs including health, has risen significantly in recent years. In the resources allocated through the budget will have added the contributions from the extraordinary oil revenues. For 2003, the nation invested about 3.4% of GDP on health, spending has increased considerably after that period, estimated in some cases increases almost 100%. Within the public health expenditure, 61% for the Ministerio del Poder Popular para la Salud, 21% to the Fondo de Salud del IVSS and the remaining 18%various contributions to health services and insurance of various government national bodies. The private insurance would not be underestimated in the country; a percentage corresponds to private insurance premiums canceled by bodies, institutions and state companies that cover their workers with such policies by collective agreements. **Free** public services: The Constitution conceives health as a right, so there is no figure of payments or copayments within the SPNS.

Table 4. Funding of Health Systems in Southern American Countries

[1] Venezuela, BR: Venezuela Bolivarian Republic denomination adopted by the country and used in international information as the World Bank statistics.

Country	GDP per capita (US$) 2014	Health spending per head (US$) 2014	Health spending rank*	Health outcomes rank*
Argentina	12,509.5	605	131	115
Brazil	11,726.8	947	127	91
Colombia	7,903.9	569	103	119
Venezuela, BR	-	873	108	106

Table 5. Per Capita Health Funding and Outcomes in South American Countries
* Among 166 countries comparison (166 = highest)

	Argentina (%)		Brazil (%)		Colombia (%)		Venezuela, BR (%)	
	Private	Public	Private	Public	Private	Public	Private	Public
2005	46.5	53.5	58.5	41.5	25.8	74.2	54.1	45.9
2006	45.3	54.7	58.2	41.8	25.8	74.2	54.2	45.8
2007	41.8	58.2	58.3	41.7	27.4	72.6	53.1	46.9
2008	38.2	61.8	56.2	43.8	29.0	71.0	69.1	30.9
2009	34.0	66.0	55.6	44.4	26.6	73.4	57.1	42.9
2010	36.4	63.6	54.2	45.8	26.4	73.6	58.5	41.5
2011	36.4	63.6	54.8	45.2	24.4	75.6	55.5	44.5
2012	41.0	59.0	55.7	44.3	23.9	76.1	65.1	34.9
2013	45.2	54.8	54.9	45.1	23.7	76.3	68.7	31.3
2014	44.6	55.4	54.0	46.0	24.9	75.1	70.7	29.3

Table 6. Private and Government expenditure on health as percentage of total expenditure on health in South American Countries2005-2014

cases of Argentina, Brazil and Colombia from 2005 to 2014. On the other hand and there is an increase in the indicator for the case of Venezuela for the same period of time.

On the other hand, for the pharmaceutical market it is important that the firms keep in mind that are the main sources of the expenditure in the health sector in the four largest markets of Southern America: Argentina, Brazil, Colombia and Venezuela, BR, as it was described in Table 6.

3.4 Pharmaceutical Markets

Although in terms of economic growth, other emerging regions such as Asia stand out more, talking about the pharmaceutical market in Latin America recorded the highest

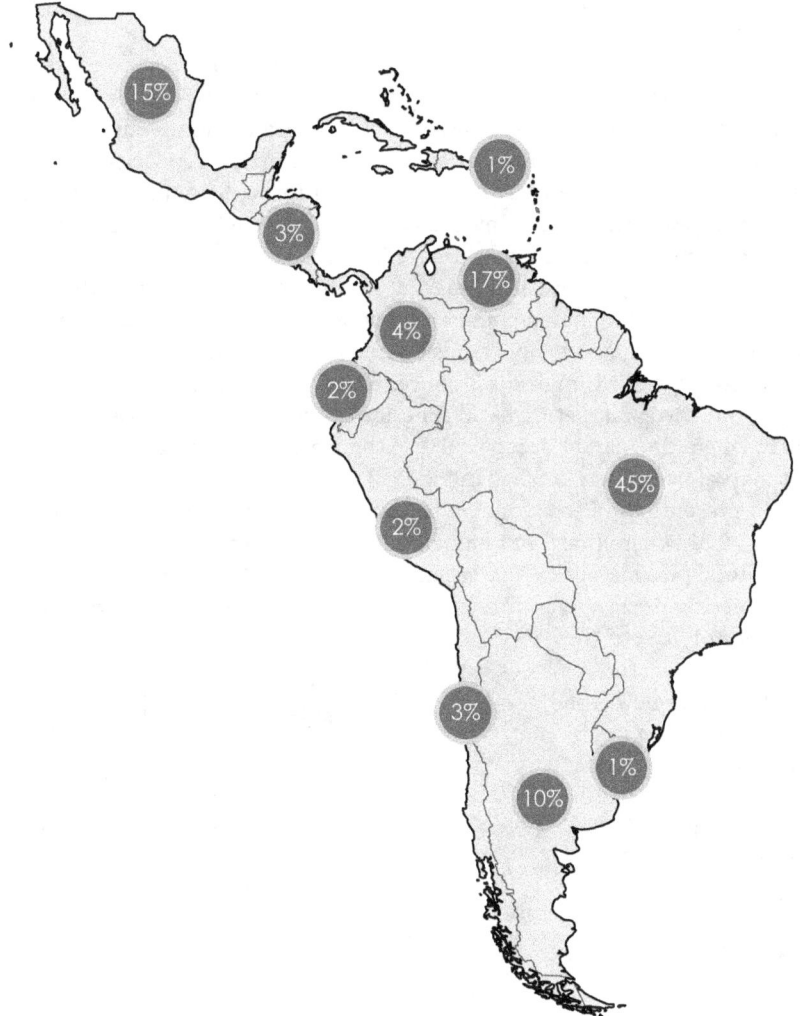

Figure 3. Percentage of Total Sales in Latin America. Years 2014 (source IMS)

growth worldwide. Phenomenon that explains why there is growing interest in investment by companies producing drugs in Southern American countries.

Something interesting is happening in the region, there is a radical change in the trend of the medicines consumed because the aging and demographic change occurs in all countries of the region. Besides, there is a steady expansion of the middle class, and it is proven that the higher middle class there is always greater consumption of drugs.

An additional factor is that in Latin America there is a lot of out-of-pocket spending; unlike Europe where they are used to having the state pay them their therapies invariably, here people buy at the pharmacy without waiting for the pay. This difference makes long recharge the industry dynamics in the payment capacity of the middle class.

The large Pharmaceutical Firms usually stationed in developed markets nowadays are not growing as expected. Hence these enterprises begin to research for new opportunities of investment in the other regions of the world, and then these firms started to increase their investment in Latin America. The growth in Latin America Pharmaceutical Markets is attracting the interests of investors either through licensing or through acquisitions. All the new activities and Investment will be affected by the regulatory matters, issues of access, price dynamics and the specific regulations.

In the case of the region of Latin America, where there is a large growth of local companies with research, development and investment. So that in many cases there are mergers, acquisitions and this somehow tends to growth and market development.

While overall spending on drugs is concentrated in the US and Europe, representing 65% of the total drug market, in Latin America is growing, as evidenced by the increase from 2010 where the market occupied 4% of the market, but these figures totaled more than 7% market by 2014 as detailed in Figure 3.

Figure 3 presents the Percentage of Total Sales of Pharmaceutical Industry in Latin America in 2014, where Brazil has had an important growth that nowadays represents 45% of the total pharmaceutical market in the region and Mexico represents 15 percent. In South America, Brazil, Argentina, Venezuela and Colombia reaches a total Percentage of Total Sales of 76% of the Pharmaceutical Industry.

In order to review the evolution of the Latin American pharmaceutical market, it was selected the variation from the December 2013 to December 2014 (fiscal year in the Southern Cone) and the results identified are presented in Table 7.

3.5 Health Technology Agencies

Nowadays, health technologies such as medicines and medical devices involve a complexity and specificity that requires an institution focused on public health,

Country	Sales 2014 (US$ Bn)	Growth (%) 2014 vs. 2013*
Brazil	23.9	4.1
Venezuela, BR	9.1	46.2
Mexico	7.5	-16.2
Argentina	5.2	-9.0
Colombia	2.1	0.1
C. America	1.5	4.2
Chile	1.6	-3.2
Ecuador	1.1	8.3
Peru	0.9	-6.6
Dominican Republic	0.5	5.3
Uruguay	0.4	-3.7
Total Latin America	53.8	4.0

Table 7. Sales and growth by country in the Latin American and Caribbean Region (source: IMS MIDAS Dec 2014 - Pharmacies Channel. Bolivia, Paraguay, Surinam and Guyana are not included in MIDAS) *Growth rates are expressed in current dollars

with an outstanding technical capacity without conflicts of interest able to implement regulations efficiently.

For most countries, the beginning of the process of drug registration began in the sixties and seventies, a period that showed a rapid increase in laws, regulations and guidelines for reporting and evaluating data regarding safety, quality and effectiveness of new health products. At that time, the pharmaceutical industry was regionalizing its operations and reaching new markets. However, the diversity of technical requirements among countries got worse the time and the costs in placing industrial products in different markets. This situation and the increase in health spending, costs in research and development and the request for new treatments tended to create a regulatory harmonization, through the creation of the Health Technology Agency (HTA), that leads those type of processes.

HTA seeks to provide health policy makers with accessible, useable and evidence-based information to guide their decisions about the appropriate use of technology and the efficient allocation of resources. HTAs also connect manufacturers with the healthcare systems. HTAs are increasingly important in Latin American countries, as this responds to the increasing industry requirements to assess the products safety, efficacy and quality as well as dealing with clinical effectiveness and cost effectiveness analysis, which constitutes the so-called "fourth hurdle" for manufacturers.

The History of HTA in Latin America

In Latin America, in the past 30 years, there have been a number of governmental and non-governmental agencies constituted for HTA review and recommendation to governments and funding agencies. The first HTA bodies in the Latin American region were created in Cuba, Mexico and Chile in 1985, followed by Brazil and Uruguay. There are different types of HTA institutions and units in Latin America, some of which are direct units of national Health Ministries as in the case of Costa Rica, Peru and Uruguay as well as other examples of in-regulatory agencies as in the case of ANVISA for Brazil and ANMAT for Argentina.

In the same way, an initiative was considered in the Pan American Region twenty years later. It was in 1999 that the Pan American Network of Pharmaceutical Harmonization (Red Pan Americana de Armonización Farmacéutica: Red-PARF) was established, then recognized in September 2000 by the 42nd Directing Council of the Pan-American Health Organization. The mission of this conference was to promote the harmonization of drug regulation in Latin America as a contribution to the quality of life and healthcare of citizens of member countries of the Pan American Health Organization (PAHO). The outcomes of this effort were the development of the Technical Guidelines, The Regulatory Processes and the strengthening of National Regulations and Agencies.

In 2011, a report of the PAHO evidenced that, although 85% of countries in Latin America have a regulatory authority, some of them show reduced abilities for drug assessment, and hence there was a lack of institutional capacity to ensure the population the access to safe and quality pharmaceutical products. The lack of harmonization, the in-

Level	Description
I	Health institutions develop some drug regulatory functions.
II	Structures and / or organization with a mandate to an RNA that meets certain regulatory functions as recommended by WHO for ensure efficacy, safety and quality of medicines.
III	A competent and efficient NRA that still needs improvements in the development of some regulatory functions as recommended by WHO for ensure efficacy, safety and quality of medicines.
IV	A competent and efficient NRA developing regulatory functions as recommended by WHO for efficacy, safety and quality of medicines. They act as reference agencies at the regional level.

Table 8. Levels for HTA Accreditation (Resolution CD50R9 PAHO)

Country	Institution	Budget (local currency)	Scope of Activities	Autonomous Agency	Monitoring Price	Pharmaco-vigilance
Argentine	ANMAT	14,7 millions	• Medicines • Cosmetics Sanitizing • Food • Medical devices	Yes	No	Yes
Brazil	ANVISA	406 millions	• Medicines Cosmetics • Food • Medical devices	Yes	Yes	Yes
Chile	ANAMED	32,2 millions	• Medicines • Cosmetics Sanitizing • Food • Medical devices • Pesticides	No	No	Yes
Colombia	INVIMA	52 millions	• Medicines • Food • Medical devices	Yes	No	Yes
México	COFEPRIS	58 millions	• Medicines • Food • Medical devices • Pesticides	Yes	NO	Yes
Perú	DIGEMID		• Medicines • Cosmetics • Medical devices	No	Yes	Yes

Table 9. Main Characteristics of Regulatory Agencies of Latin America and the Caribbean

adequate professional expertise of examiners and the reduce quality of the control laboratories in the region appear to be the main reason for inadequate abilities for drug evaluation. One of the aims of PAHO is assisting countries in regulatory issues such as evaluation of regulatory capabilities and building up skills in this area. For this purpose the PAHO carried out an evaluation proposing indicators to assess National Regulatory Systems (NRS), National Regulatory Authority (NRA), Marketing Authorizations (MA), Manufacturers Authorizations (LM), Pharmacovigilance (PV), Clinical Trials (CT), Good Manufacturing Practice (GMP), quality control laboratories and Market Surveillance (MS). These indicators were tabulated and the compliance limits defined levels relative to a reference agency proposed by Organización Panamericana de la Salud (OPS). The taxonomy was established based on the parameters shown in Table 8.

Among the Latin American countries, Chile's Instituto de Salud Pública (ISP) sets at Level III. Argentina, Colombia, Brazil and Cuba have already reached Level IV.

Most of the countries in the Region have Regulatory Agencies, some of them are an independent body like ANVISA (Brazil), INVIMA (Colombia) or ANMAT (Argentina). In other cases, they belong to the Ministry of Health, but they have relative autonomy as the "Instituto Izquieta Perez" in Ecuador, DIGEMID (Dirección General de Medicamentos, Insumos y Drogas) in Perù and Departamento de Control Nacional del Instituto de Salud Pública of Chile. In some other countries have adopted a different organizational form: the Regulatory Authority is created as a department or area of the Ministry of Health, as it happens in Dominican Republic (Dirección General de Drogas y Farmacias), Paraguay (Dirección Nacional de Vigilancia Sanitaria) and Uruguay (División de Productos de Salud). Despite most countries have legislation that enables surveillance and control by the authorities, the legislation is considered by PAHO very weak throughout the region. As a consequence, to have updated and harmonized regulation is an important requirement, but not enough in order to correct pharmaceutical market failures.

In Table 9 is shown the main aspects of the Regulatory Agencies in selected countries of Latin America and the Caribbean.

Red ETSA – Pan-American Health Organization (PAHO/WHO)

A new HTA evaluation commission to monitor the activities of national HTAs on a regional level was created in 2010 under the name Red ETSA. The commission officially came into force in June 2011, with 13 members affiliated including Argentina, Bolivia, Brazil, Canada, Chile, Colombia, Costa Rica, Cuba, Ecuador, México, Paraguay, Peru, and Uruguay. The commission is part of the Pan American Health organization (PAHO) and is funded for 4 years as a result of a grant agreement between PAHO and the Brazilian health commission ANVISA. 22 international institutions are currently members of Red ETSA. The resolution CSP28.R9 on the Assessment and Incorporation of Health Technologies in the healthcare systems in Latin America, created in September 2012, is the first HTA related resolution supported by the whole Latin American region. This resolution has been a hit in the region, and is approved by PAHO and agreed by the overall Red ETSA network. These are the aims of the resolution:

- Integration of HTA in public policies related to health technologies;
- Implementation of an institutional framework for decision making processes based on HTA;
- Reinforcement of human resources;
- Promotion of evidence generation and information diffusion;
- Rational use of health technologies;
- Promotion of networking.

How the future looks?

The two countries that have seen the most dramatic impact from regional improvements in the field of HTA are Brazil and Uruguay. In the case of Brazil, through national and inter regional collaboration, the country has achieved improved collaborations between the national HTA CONITEC and ANVISA in terms of producing systematic reviews, economic evaluation, budget impact assessment, and HTA reports. HTA reports have been especially beneficial to lower the prices of drugs in the country since Brazil has some of the highest prices in the region. The set-up of Colombia's new HTA IETS is also expected to have a conspicuous influence on pricing policies in the country. So far, Brazil, Uruguay and Colombia are the countries with highest HTA influences in the region at present, with Mexico having a lesser degree of influence and Chile going under a restructuring of its HTA system but with potential of building strong HTA competencies in the medium term.

From an international perspective, HTAs in Latin America are mainly influenced by the Spanish tradition of regional HTA agencies and by the international agency of HTA of the UK National Institute for Clinical Excellence. Nevertheless, European agencies are most likely to influence Latin American HTAs in terms of safety and clinical effectiveness decisions while cost effectiveness analysis is entirely country specific.

3.6 Market access

There is no 'one size fits all' approach to Market access in Latin America — while it is an attractive region overall for pharmaceutical industry, each country is unique and companies must tailor their approach and be sensitive to national characteristics and variations among countries.

There are significant differences in pricing and reimbursement across the region. Some countries, such as the region's large emerging economy of Brazil, utilize HTA assessment for pricing, while others such as Mexico use reference prices; others (e.g. Chile and Argentina) leave it to the companies to decide price. However, the landscape is dynamic and needs monitoring, with Colombia as one example transitioning from free pricing to reference pricing.

In terms of reimbursement, there is a wide range of payers — from health plans and insurers, to hospital financial management and health department officials — all trying to find a balance between the need for cost-containment and increased consumer expectations for improved healthcare.

In countries with high levels of private payer autonomy — e.g. Brazil and Mexico circled here in cluster 1 — private payers are free to decide which drugs they reimburse in any of the multiple health plans they offer. In countries with a low level of private payer autonomy — e.g. Colombia and Chile in cluster 2 — the private payers have a reduced level of freedom regarding funding decisions. In Colombia for example, the contributive EPS — the Health Maintenance Organization (HMO) segment, which subcontracts mostly to private providers — needs to reimburse all drugs on the national health formulary (POS). Now this national formulary does not include most premium drugs, but with the upcoming healthcare reform, this could change.

The level of access of those with private coverage is also an important consideration. Firstly, access to both public and private hospitals gives physicians in public institutions access to, and experience with, patients taking premium, innovative medicines. Secondly, it usually means that the private sector has more freedom in making coverage decisions as the citizen is already covered by a national health insurance.

Mexico

The private sector in Mexico has a limited patient base — only 3.5% of population — but provides a relevant benchmark in terms of early product adoption and purchasing power.

Private payers can be divided into two segments — "normal" private insurances and HMOs. Unlike "normal" private insurances, HMOs have non-mandatory formularies, where selected premium drugs (over $10,000) can be included. However, since 2012, all private and HMO insurances carry one-time and usually non-renewable policy limits. Depending on the policy these limits can be prohibitive for the use of premium innovative drugs. In addition, there is a smaller segment of patients seen in private hospitals who are very wealthy individuals (often "health tourists") who pay "out-of-pocket" for products prescribed by their treating physician.

On the public sector side, most premium innovative drugs are classified as "clave 5000" and their prescription is rare outside certain specialist hospitals. The few granted access now have to face extra layers of approval before reaching the hands of doctors — the two major public payers (IMSS and ISSTE), have both recently introduced a new prescription control program (called Catálogo II at IMSS), which restricts and delays access to premium innovative drugs by up to three weeks due to a centralized pre-authorization and drug delivery process.

Colombia

Colombia currently has near-universal coverage, something rarely seen in Latin America. The financial strain however, has created the need for change, and the country is entering a period of transformation. Currently, Colombia's health system operates under two schemes; contributory and subsidized. Forty percent of the Colombian population holds formal employment and receives health insurance through the contributory scheme, granting access to private hospitals. The remaining 60% of the population are subsidized by the public health system. The greatest potential for premium in-patient drugs lies within the contributive EPS. This is because the use of premium drugs is higher in private than in public hospitals due to their increased purchasing power, their strong negotiation power, and the existence of independent funding, if the hospital has the status of a foundation with independent resources.

The contributive market is currently fragmented into 21 players (some of them also offering subsidized insurances). A key factor differentiating Colombia from other Latin American markets is this de-centralization of key customers over the country. Being successful in Colombia means being able to adapt to this structural and geographical reality. Premium innovative drugs are usually excluded from the national compulsory health plan (POS). In order to prescribe a non-POS drug, the hospital needs to send a request to the EPS in charge of the patient — this is either authorized and reimbursed, or rejected. Although the cost for the drug is not borne by the EPS, they have incentives not to approve non-POS treatments.

However, two major changes proposed in the healthcare reforms are imminent — firstly the abolition of funding for non-listed treatments, and secondly the creation of a unique national fund for direct hospital financing. The implementation of a unique benefit package (Mi Plan) is expected to represent an additional market access hurdle.

Access to Mexico

To achieve hospital access in Mexico, try to facilitate the use of your product in reference institutions, which can be both private and public (e.g. tertiary care IMSS hospitals). Doctors who use of that product and work across both settings can be powerful advocates. One may also consider organizing medical education programs in partnership with the reference institutions, and establish preceptor ship programs for other doctors to visit reference hospitals. However, it is important that key account managers are in place on the ground to liaise with individual physicians about the benefits of the product, as protocols are only loosely followed in private hospitals.

Access to Colombia

In Colombia, a discount pricing agreement may be essential to incentivize the hospital to include a product in the formulary, and this may include portfolio agreements and Managed Entry Agreements. In the case of an acute care drug, it is advisable to avoid pre-clearance and instead facilitate approval post-use by facilitating supportive clinical and health economical evidence for your product and implementing medical education of prescribers to ensure correct and rapid patient identification. To help achieve formulary inclusion you should build KOL and medical society endorsement and consider investing in local cost-effectiveness and cost-benefit studies. Make sure you map the budgeting process in the different hospitals in order to identify the key stakeholders, and then support them with a budget forecast tool as well as with a business case for your product.

7 Final Comments

Based in the analyses developed in this chapter, many Southern American Countries are trying to introduce reference pricing and other price control tools in order to keep track of the expenditure in drugs. Instead of that situation at least one of the main analysts of the sector is predicting an increase in the Compounded Average Growth Rate (CAGR) for the period 2014-2019, as it is detailed in Figure 4.

As a concluding remark of this chapter it is suggested that the assumptions adopted by the consultants and the industry, to estimate the projected rate of growth of the Pharmaceutical Sector, should be carefullyr eviewed in order to include the effects of the new public policies and instruments developed in the region, like HTA and Reference Pricing.

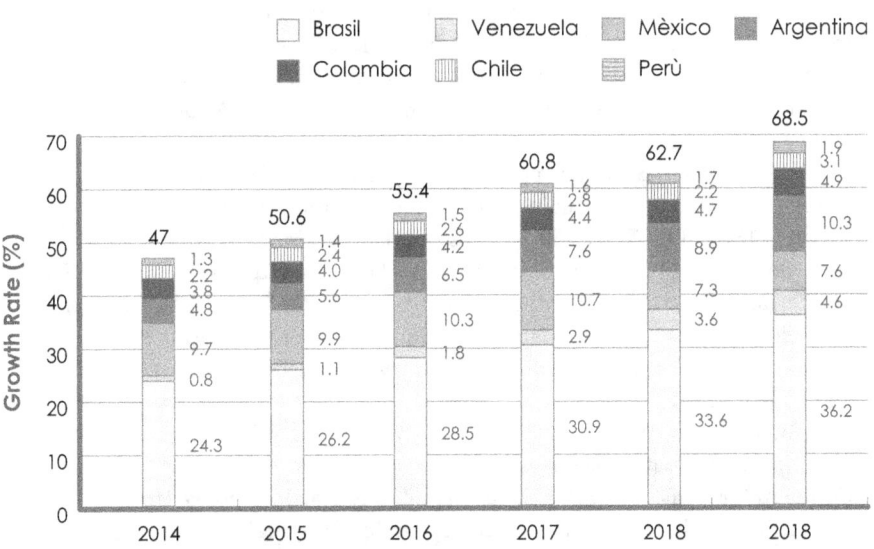

Figure 4. Projected growth in major countries in the region (US$ Billion). Exchange rate: Bloomberg.com (May 4th 2015), except Argentina and Venezuela, BR. Argentine exchange rate 35%, below official rate. Venezuelan rate is 90% below the official. Growth region would be 18% in case official rates of these countries would be used. Ex - man price MIDAS. Rebate not included. It includes audited channels and not audited. Central America, Caribe, Paraguay, Uruguay, Bolivia and Ecuador are not included (Source: IMS Market Prognosis, Q1 2015)

3.8 **To know more**

- Administración Nacional de Medicamentos, Alimentos y Tecnología Médica – ANMAT. Available at www.anmat.gov.ar/
- Agência Nacional de Vigilância Sanitária – ANViSa. Available at http://portal.anvisa.gov.br/
- Aitken M. El mercado farmacéutico mundial: Dinámica y Perspectivas. IMS World Review Conference 2015. Available at http://imsworldreview.com/2015/descargas/ AR-IWR2015-MurrayAitken.pdf (last accessed September 2016)
- Augustovski F, Diaz Rojas JA, Bosi Ferraz M, et al. Status Update of the Reimbursement Review Environment in the Public Sector across Four Latin American Countries. *Value In Health Regional Issues* 2012; 1: 223-7
- Augustovski F, Iglesias C, Manca A, et al, Barriers to Generalizability of Health Economic Evaluations in Latin America and the Caribbean Region. *Pharmacoeconomics* 2009; 27: 919-29
- Bellanger M, Picon P, Stuwe L. Una Mirada sobre la evaluación de las tecnologías de la salud en Brasil. *News Across Latin America* 2015; 3
- Boutayeb A. The double burden of communicable and non-communicable diseases in developing countries. *Trans R Soc Trop Med Hyg* 2006; 100: 191-9
- Center For Global Development – CGDev. Available at www.cgdev.org/
- Centre for Reviews and Dissemination. University of York. Available at http://www.york.ac.uk/crd/
- CEPAL – Comisión Económica para América Latina. Panorama Social de América Latina. 2015. Available at http://repositorio.cepal.org/bitstream/ handle/11362/39965/1/S1600227_es.pdf (last accessed September 2016)
- Chowdhury CA, Martin de Bustamante M. HTA or Reference pricing? The Future of Pharmaceutical Cost Controls in Latin America. Workshop ISPOR, Santiago de Chile, 2015. Available at http://www.ispor.org/conferences/Mexico0911/ presentations/W12-Bustamante-Chowdhury-ALLSLIDES.pdf (last accessed September 2016)
- Comisión Federal Para La Protección Contra Riesgos Sanitarios – COFEPRIS. Available at www.cofepris.gob.mx
- Cunha AM, Magalhães Prates D, Ferrari-Filho F. Brazil Responses to the Global Financial Crisis: a well succeed example of Keynesian policies? *Panoeconomicus* 2011; 5: 693-714. Available at http://www.panoeconomicus.rs/ casopis/2011_5/07_Andre_Moreira_Cunha.pdf (last accessed September 2016)
- Díaz C. Gestión de Servicios Asistenciales: ¿Cómo convertir un Jefe de Servicio en un Gerente? Buenos Aires: Ediciones ISALUD, 2009
- Dirección General de Medicamentos, Insumos y Drogas – DiGeMID. Available at www.digemid.minsa.gob.pe/

- Drummond MF, Schwartz JS, Johnson B, et al. Key principles for the improved conduct of health technology assessments for resource allocation decisions. *Int J Technol Assess Health Care* 2008; 24: 244-58
- Drummond MF, Sculpher MJ, Torrance G, et al. Methods for the Economic Evaluation of Health Care Programmes. (3rd ed.) New York : Oxford University Press, 2005
- Fondo Nacional de Recursos – FNR. Miradas externas sobre el FNR: Estudio de Factum sobre percepción de imagen del FNR en la Opinión Pública, en médicos, periodistas y operadores políticos. Montevideo, 2011. Available at http://www.fnr.gub.uy/sites/default/files/publicaciones/FNR_miradas_externas.pdf (last accessed September 2016)
- Glanc M. Modelos de Asociación Público Privada en el Desarrollo de Hospitales Públicos de America Latina. Buenos Aires: Ed. Isalud, 2015
- Glassman A, Zoloa JI. How Much Will Health Coverage Cost? Future Health Spending Scenarios in Brazil, Chile, and Mexico, Working Paper 382, Center for Global Development, Washington, 2014. Available at http://www.cgdev.org/sites/default/files/CGD-Working-Paper-382-Glassman-Zoloa-future-health-spending-Latin-America.pdf (last accessed September 2016)
- González García G, De la Puente y Tarragona S. Medicamentos: Salud, Política y Economía. Buenos Aires: Ed. Isalud, 2005
- González García G. Salud para los argentinos: economía, política y reforma del sistema de salud en Argentina. Buenos Aires: Ed. Isalud, 2004
- Health Technology Assessment International – HTAi. Available at http://www.htai.org/
- Homedes N, Ugalde C. Improving access to pharmaceuticals in Brazil and Argentina. *Health Policy and Planning* 2006; 21: 123-31
- Homedes N, Ugalde C. Multisource drug policies in Latin America: survey of 10 countries. Bulletin of the World Health Organization 2005; 83: 1-80
- Husereau D, Drummond M, Petrou S, et al.; ISPOR Health Economic Evaluation Publication Guidelines-CHEERS Good Reporting Practices Task Force. Consolidated Health Economic Evaluation Reporting Standards (CHEERS)--explanation and elaboration: a report of the ISPOR Health Economic Evaluation Publication Guidelines Good Reporting Practices Task Force. *Value Health* 2013; 16: 231-50
- Iglesias C, Drummond M, Rovira J; NEVALAT Project Group. Health care decision making processes in Latin America: Problems and prospects for the use of economic evaluation. *Int J Technol Assess Health Care* 2005; 21: 1-14
- IMS Consulting Group P&MA, Pricing & Market Access Outlook Edition 2015/2016.
- IMS Health. Available at www.imshealth.com
- Instituto de Salud Pública de Chile – ISPCH. Available at http://www.ispch.cl/anamed
- Instituto Nacional de Vigilancia de Medicamentos y Alimentos – INVIMA. Available at https://www.invima.gov.co/

- International Development Research Centre – IDRC. Aiming for equity in Colombia's health system reform: Achievements and continuing challenges: International Development Research Centre, 2008
- International Society for Pharmacoeconomics and Outcomes Research – ISPOR. Available at www.ispor.org
- ISAGS, UNASUR. Sistemas de Salud en Suramérica, desafíos para la universalidad, la integralidad y la equidad. Río de Janeiro: Instituto Suramericano de Gobierno en Salud (ISAGS), 2012. Available at http://www.cridlac.org/digitalizacion/pdf/spa/doc19134/doc19134-contenido.pdf (last accessed September 2016)
- ISAGS, UNASUR. Sistemas de Salud en Suramérica: desafíos para la universalidad, la integralidad y la equidad. Rio de Janeir: ISAGS, 2012. Available at http://www.isags-unasur.org/uploads/biblioteca/2/bb[8]ling[2]anx[9].pdf (last accessed September 2016)
- Laranjeira FO, Petramale CA. A avaliação econômica em saúde na tomada de decisão: a experiência da CONITEC. *BIS Bol Inst Saúde Impresso* 2012; 14: 165-70
- Lemgruber A, Santfelices Cuevas E, Alfonso R, et al. Pharmacoeconomics and Outcomes Research in Latin America - Argentina, Brazil, Chile, Colombia, and México. ISPOR 1st Latin America Conference. Cartagena, 2007
- McGhan WF, Al M, Doshi JA, et al. The ISPOR Good Practices for Quality Improvement of Cost - Effectiveness Research Task Force Report. Value Health 2009; 12:1086 - 99.
- Ministério da Saúde. Secretaria de Ciência, Tecnologia e Insumos Estratégicos. Departamento de Ciência e Tecnologia. Diretrizes metodológicas: Diretriz de Avaliação Econômica. Ed 2°. Brasília: Ministério da Saúde, 2014. Available at http://bvsms.saude.gov.br/bvs/publicacoes/diretrizes_metodologicas_diretriz_avaliacao_economica.pdf (last accessed September 2016)
- Nicholls A, Pannelay A. Health Outcomes and Costs: A 166-country comparison. The Economist Intelligence Unit, 2014. Available at http://stateofreform.com/wp-content/uploads/2015/11/Healthcare-outcomes-index-2014.pdf (last accessed September 2016)
- Nuijten C, Pronk MH, Brorens MJA, et al. Reporting format for economic evaluation, part II: focus on modelling studies. *Pharmacoeconomics* 1998; 14: 259-68
- Oortwijn W, Mathijssen J, Banta D. The role of health technology assessment on pharmaceutical reimbursement in selected middle-income countries. *Health Policy* 2010; 95: 174-184
- Organización Panamericana de la Salud –OPS/ Organización Mundial de la Salud – OMS. El acceso a los medicamentos de alto costo en las Américas. Contexto, desafíos y perspectivas. Washington DC: OPS/OMS, 2009
- Outterson K. Pharmaceutical Arbitrage: Balancing Access and Innovation in International Prescription Drug Markets. *Yale J Health Policy Law Ethics* 2005; 5: 193-291
- PAHO – Pan American Health Organization. Available at www.paho.org/hq/

- Payne K, Annemans L. Reflections on Market Access for Personalized Medicine: Recommendations for Europe. *Value In Health* 2013; 16: S32-8
- Pichon-Riviere A, Augustovski F, Rubinstein A. Health Technology Assessment in Argentina: six years in perspective. 3rd Annual Meeting Health Technology Assessment International – HTAi .Adelaide, 2006
- Quintiles. Available at www.quintiles.com
- Resolution CSP28.R9. Health technology assessment and incorporation Into health systems. The 28th Pan American Sanitary Conference. Washington, D.C 17-21 September 2012
- Rubinstein A, Belizán M, Discacciati V. Are economic evaluations and health technology assessments increasingly demanded in times of rationing health services? The case of the Argentine financial crisis. *Int J Technol Assess Health Care* 2007; 23: 169-76
- Santa María, JM. Dinámicas y Perspectivas del Mercado Farmacéutico en América Latina y Argentina. IMS World Review Conference, 2015. Available at http://imsworldreview.com/2015/descargas/AR-IWR2015-JuanManuelSantaMaria.pdf (last accessed September 2016)
- Schiavone MA, Ríos J. Economía y Financiamiento de la Salud. Buenos Aires: Ed. Dunken, 2013
- Schweiger A, De la Puente C. Sistema de Información Gerencial como base del presupuesto por resultados y Costos en Hospitales públicos seleccionados. Buenos Aires: Comisión Nacional de Salud Investiga, 2008
- Schweiger A, San Martin M, Levcovich M. Il Deficit nel Sistema Sanitario Argentino e analisi degli strumenti di copertura. In: Rapporto CEIS –Sanità: Il Governo del Sistema Sanitario. Roma, CEIS, 2006
- Schweiger A. Moving towards Universal Health Coverage. A review of Argentina and Uruguay cases. IHEA presentation, Milan, 2015
- Skaltsa K. The challenges of introducing HTA in Latin America. HTA Uncovered 2014; 5: 1-8. Available at http://www.quintiles.com/~/media/library/fact%20 sheets/hta-uncovered-may-2014.pdf (last accessed September 2016)
- Strapp Jr J, Walker J, Fromer L. Emerging Payment Models. Navigate the current state of financial uncertainty to prepare for the future of health care spending. Eyeforpharma, 2016. Available at http://thekinetixgroup.com/wp-content/ uploads/2016/02/Emerging-Payment-Models-Whitepaper.pdf (last accessed September 2016)
- The World Bank website 2016. Available at http://data.worldbank.org/
- Tobar F. Cambios en el paradigma en Salud Pública. Buenos Aires: XII Congreso de CLAD, 2008. Last accessed http://www.federicotobar.com.ar/nf_pdf5/Cambios.pdf (last accessed September 2016)
- Torres R, González Prieto G. Una Contribución a la Sustentabilidad del Sistema de Salud: Propuesta de Mejora de Cuidados de ECNT-DP. Buenos Aires: Ed. Isalud, 2016
- Torres R. Política sanitaria en el país de los argentinos. Reflexiones para el día después. Buenos Aires: Ed. Isalud, 2015

- UNASUR – Unión de Naciones Suramericanas. Available at http://www.unasursg.org/
- UNCTAD – United Nations Conference on Trade and Development Available at http://unctad.org/en/Pages/Home.aspx
- Walker D, Wilson R, Sharma R, et al. Best Practices for Conducting Economic Evaluations in Health Care: A Systematic Review of Quality Assessment Tools. Rockville (MD): Agency for Healthcare Research and Quality (US), 2012
- World Health Organization – WHO. Health Accounts. Available at www.who.int/health-accounts/en/

Market Access in South Eastern Europe Countries

Tarik Čatić

Introduction

This chapter will provide an overview of health care system financing with a special focus on medicines pricing and reimbursement in selected countries of South Eastern Europe. Countries healthcare systems explained include former Yugoslavia countries and Albania, which are passing a transition period in the last twenty years after being granted independence in the early 1990s.

After World War II, from 1945 Yugoslavia was recreated as Socialist state consisted of six republics (Bosnia-Herzegovina, Croatia, Macedonia, Montenegro, Serbia, and Slovenia) and two autonomous provinces (Kosovo and Vojvodina as part of Serbia) [1].

In 1991 Yugoslavia was dimished when Slovenia and Croatia declared its independence. In 1992 the further declarations of independence by two other republics, Macedonia, as well as Bosnia and Herzegovina, left only Serbia and Montenegro within Yugoslavia until 2006 when Montenegro declared its independence and when the Yugoslavian federation was finally ended [2].

Figure 1 represents the geographical structure of this region after the disintegration process finished as of 2008.

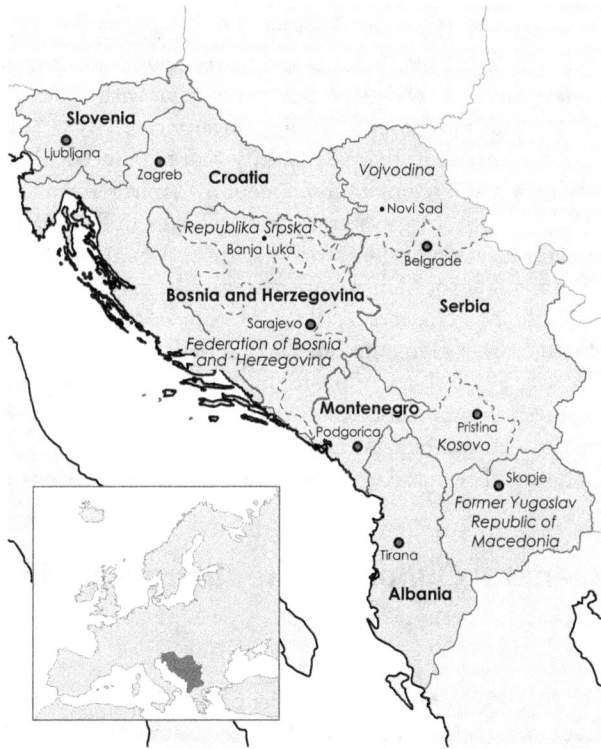

Figure 1. Former Yugoslavia as of January 2008 [2]

Slovenia and Croatia became members of European Union, while other countries are implementing reform and are in the process of joining.

Historical influence and heritage of healthcare sector

The former socialist Yugoslavia's healthcare system was unique among the European socialist countries in terms of financing, as it was financed through a compulsory social insurance (kind of Bismarck Model), but the access to healthcare was a constitutional right of all citizens. However, the provision of service was more like in the Semashko model, with physicians as salaried state employees [3].

Healthcare system in former Yugoslavia was unique among Easter Europe countries based on so-called Stampar model and was funded from compulsory social insurance contribution. After country dissolution, most of the newly independent countries kept this system and introduced some new laws related to healthcare regulation introducing a private sector, especially in the field of medicine, dentistry, pharmacies and laboratories.

Albania, as another country which will be covered in this chapter, has Soviet Semashko model of healthcare financing, meaning that central government budget finance healthcare. From 1995 Albania has introduced health insurance which does not play an important role as in other countries in this region [4].

In general, the health system is financed by public health insurance funds which collect insurance contributions and finance public healthcare institutions mainly, but sometimes private as well, through contracting with them. So public health insurance funds are the only purchaser of healthcare services.

All countries in the past twenty years are faced with different problems in financing healthcare and trying to implement different reforms in order to assure sustainable and efficient healthcare system. Latest reforms in the healthcare sector, in general, brought decentralization of the system in case of Albania, Bulgaria, Croatia and Romania, and development of social insurance systems like in Albania, Bulgaria, Croatia, Former Yugoslav Republic of Macedonia – FYROM, Slovenia, and Romania. Some countries had introduced market elements especially in the field of primary healthcare (Albania, Bulgaria, Croatia, FYROM, and Slovenia) establishing family physician practices [5]. In Table 1 is reported a classification of countries based on income group [6], while in Table 2 is shown pharmaceutical expenditure in 2005 in Western Balkan which is more or less kept the same trend even today in terms of percentage relations among countries [7].

4.2 General Outlook of Healthcare System and Health Policies

Albania

The major funder and provider of healthcare services in Albania is Ministry of Health. Even reorganized it still continue to assume the lead role in most areas of healthcare in this country.

Country Name	Country Code	Income Group	Special Notes
Albania	ALB	Upper middle income	
Bosnia and Herzegovina	BIH	Upper middle income	Based on official government statistics for chain linked series; the new reference year is 2010.
Kosovo		Lower middle income	Kosovo became a World Bank member on June 29, 2009. Since 1999, Kosovo has been a territory under international administration pursuant to UN Security Council Resolution 1244 (1999).
Macedonia	MKD	Upper middle income	New base year is 2005.
Montenegro	MNE	Upper middle income	Montenegro declared independence in 2006. Where available, data for each country are shown separately. However, for Serbia, some indicators continue to include data for Montenegro through 2005.
Serbia	SRB	Upper middle income	When possible data for Serbia are separated from Montenegro since its independance from 2006. For Kosovo, from 2009 data are separately presented and analysed due to geo-political changes and statistics reported for Kosovo to World Bank from 2009.

Table 1. Income group of countries by World Bank Classification [6]

	Albania	Bosnia & Herzegovina	Macedo-nia	Montene-gro	Serbia	Kosovo
Total pharma-ceutical expendi-ture = market size (USD million)	93*	180	130	39	450	65-80
Market growth rate local currency (%)	>10	10-15	NA	15	20	10
Total pharmaceutical spending° (%)	32	12.4	8-15	14.9	14.8	30
Drug expenditure per capita (USD)	26.5	<50	65	65	60	33-40

Table 2. Pharmaceutical market overview in Western Balkan countries [7]
* 2004
° Including out-of-pocket payments, as a % of health care expenditure

It "owns" most health services, with the partial exception of primary care. Albanian health services are funded through a mix of taxation and statutory insurance. The majority of funding comes from the state budget, but the tax base is problematic due to low incomes, the large informal economy and problems with tax collection. The introduction of social health insurance in 1995 represent major structural reform in Albania. From 1996 Health Insurance Institute (HII) became autonomous as national statutory fund and is responsible for governing health funds [8].

The public healthcare system offers primary ambulatory healthcare and hospital care (secondary and tertiary services).

The primary ambulatory healthcare centers offer the following services:

- Adults healthcare. Main diagnosis and treatments by the family doctors for the prevalent diseases among the adults like hypertension, diabetes, angina, cardiac insufficiency, anaemia, asthma, depression, infection of respiratory paths, skin problems, arthritis etc.
- Children healthcare. Monitoring of growing and development, diagnosis and treatment of pediatric health problems, information and education for preventing the prevalent diseases among children, vaccination, etc.
- Women's health and reproductive healthcare. Clinical diagnosis and treatment during pregnancy, HIV/syphilis's test, hepatitis B test, etc.
- Emergency healthcare. The initial management and stabilization of urgent problems, asthma attacks, chest pains, fractures, wounds and scratches care.
- Minimum laboratory tests. Urine analysis, glucosemia, pregnancy test, vaginal secretions analysis.

University and Regional Public Hospitals offer diagnosis and treatment in a wide varietUniversity and Regional Public Hospitals offer diagnosis and treatment in a wide variety of medical specialties, emergency cases, analytic laboratories, imagery services, unique tertiary services such as MRI, Scanner, Mammography, Angiography, Coronarography, Fibrogastroscopy, Fibrocolonoscopy, Scintigraphy, etc. In the public insurance scheme are included even some private hospitals which are contracted by The Fund for some services that the public sector cannot provide for all the population, such as dialysis, coronary angioplasty, coronary angiography, definitive pacemaker implant, aorta-coronary bypass, valve intervention, congenital intervention, renal transplant and cochlear transplant.

Part of the public healthcare insurance is the drugs reimbursement list (RL), which is published each year and includes the drugs that are fully covered by the insurance or offered with co-payment. Patient co-payments are mainly applicable to outpatient services and pharmaceuticals and are kept at a low level. Due to pharmacy privatization process medicine prices has increased but the effect to patient has been mitigated by health insurance subsidies especially for essential drugs. Pharmaceuticals included into the essential list are fully or partly reimbursed, while other drugs, most dental care, and some other services are paid for out-of-pocket. The co-payment is also applied to the drugs in the RL. Only the first alternative is fully covered by The Fund for the categories: retired, children aged 0-12 months, disabled persons, war invalid, veterans, people suffering from tuberculosis and cancer, blind people, orphans, people suffering thalassemia major, multiple sclerosis, people who had a renal transplant; for the other alternatives the patient has to co-pay the difference in price (price of the alternative chosen – price of the first alternative in the list).

For the other categories of insured people: woman in maternity leave, unemployed, active, children 1-14 years old, students from 14-25 years old, partially disabled (gr. III, IV), voluntary self-insured; only the 50% of the price of the first alternative in the reimbursed list, is covered by The Fund.

The private healthcare sector is developing rapidly the recent years. The facilities of this sector can offer from primary to tertiary services. Part of the private sector is even the pharmaceutical service. The Fund contracts the private pharmacies in order to offer to the patients the drugs included in the RL.

Bosnia and Herzegovina

Among all Western Balkan countries, Bosnia and Herzegovina have the most complicated organization which is also reflected healthcare system financing and medicines reimbursement. Dayton peace agreement which ended war activities in Bosnia and Herzegovina in 1995 set administrative parts of the country: Federation of Bosnia and Herzegovina consisted of 10 cantons, entity Republic of Srpska and Brcko District. This structure reflects on the health system and its financing.

The Ministry of Civil Affairs on a state level deal with the health system in terms of coordination between entities and international relationships [9]. It is also responsible for establishing Agency for medicines and medical devices of Bosnia and Herzegovina (ALMBiH). This institution has unified pharmaceutical market in terms of marketing authorization. Also, the intention of ALMBiH is to introduce medicines price control mechanism through referral pricing system (referral countries Serbia, Slovenia, Croatia, and additionally Austria and Italy in case-referent product is not available in primary referral countries). Even Rulebook on price regulation is appointed in 2011; it is still not effective due to political issues on entity level [10]. Key players are ministries of health on the entity and cantonal levels.

Kosovo

The health system in Kosovo was mainly based on the *Semashko* model of healthcare delivery. The central government is the purchaser and provider of healthcare services. Healthcare is financed by taxes collected through Kosovo budget as well as municipal budgets and direct payments.

In 2009 the total health expenditure in Kosovo was € 158.22 million. A large proportion of total healthcare spending in Kosovo, however, occurs outside of the budget, in the form of out-of-pocket payments by private individuals [11].

Since Kosovo is recently formed country health system is not fully developed. Key healthcare related bodies are:

- Ministry Of Health. It creates and implements the policies of the health system. Health expenditure for the year 2015 was 120 mil € only 2% increase from previous year. The budget for drug consumption and medical devices around 40 mill€.
- Kosovo Medicines Agency. It functions as a branch of the Ministry of Health and is responsible for the Regulatory-Marketing Authorization of Medicinal Products as well is responsible for the import licenses. According to the regulations, the time of issuing a marketing authorization certificate is 210 days from the day of application.
- Fund for Health Insurance. Still not functional. According to the Law on Healthcare, Fund for Health Insurance is designated as an institution but will be operational within 3 years.

Healthcare services are provided by public, private and public-private healthcare institutions. The public sector includes primary care (177 Family Medicine Centers), secondary hospital service (7 regional hospitals), and tertiary hospital (University Clinical Center of Kosovo) while the private sector covers pharmaceutical service (totally private, except the hospital pharmacies), dental services, diagnostic clinics, and private hospitals.

Macedonia, FYR

The Republic of Macedonia, situated in the middle of the Balkan peninsula, has gained independence in 1991. The country has gone through a number of healthcare reforms in recent years. The healthcare system in the Republic of Macedonia is organized on three levels: primary, secondary and tertiary level.

The Ministry of Health's core functions focus on health policy formulation and implementation, priority-setting and monitoring of the health system's performance and this Ministry is accountable to the Government according to the Law in Healthcare. The Health Insurance Fund (HIF) is an independent institution which provides most of the financial resources required for the health system functioning. The healthcare insurance is determined by the Law on Health Care Insurance. This law was passed by the Parliament of the Republic of Macedonia in 2000. It regulates the healthcare insurance for the citizens, the rights and the obligations of participants in the healthcare insurance, as well as the health insurance model, which is mandatory and voluntary in the Republic of Macedonia. Health insurance is based on principles of comprehensiveness, solidarity, equity and effective use of resources covering almost entire population.

Since 1994 co-payment scheme has been introduced in order to control overconsumption in the healthcare system. This scheme provides additional revenues to the healthcare organizations through direct payment by uninsured persons or for providing services that are not included into the basic beneficiary package.

Key players and decision maker in Macedonia are Ministry of Health and Health Insurance Fund (HIF). The HIF determines the reference price of the drugs, medical supplies, equipment, orthopedic materials and others remedial supplies and spending materials which are used in the healthcare of the insurers which HIF reimburses and the minister gives approval.

Montenegro

Montenegro is the smallest market with the very small population. Healthcare system is financed through contributions for health insurance that is being collected in the Republic fund for health insurance and paid to health institutions for provided services to its beneficiaries [12]. For individuals that have no health insurance, the financial means are provided from the state budget of the Republic of Montenegro. The 30% of total health expenditure goes to pharmaceuticals and medical devices. Total pharmaceutical expenditure in 2014 was around 62,3 million € and have increasing trends despite government recommendation on cost savings. Healthcare system is organized like in other ex-Yugoslavia countries through primary (ambulatory care) secondary and tertiary level (hospitals and clinical center).

Serbia

Serbia, like other parts of former Yugoslavia, has inherited a health system financed by compulsory health insurance contributions, based on payroll taxes. The system was used to provide easy access to comprehensive health services for all population.

Healthcare in Serbia is provided through a wide network of public healthcare institutions owned and controlled by the Ministry of Health, but also private sector is in expansion. The private sector is excluded from public funding. In Serbia, there is no supplementary component of the public sector and there is no additional, supplementary, parallel private health insurance which could enrich the existing scarce financial resources of the system. The private provision of healthcare services, although limited, is on the rise, particularly in certain areas, such as dentistry [13].

In principle, insurance coverage is provided to all employed persons, pensioners, and self-employed people and farmers who are contributor payers, including the spouse, dependent children and elderly parents of an insurer.

The most important source of healthcare financing in Serbia is the Republic Health Insurance Fund (RHIF) [14]. RHIF is financed also with supplementary financing from various budgetary sources, such as Pension Fund, Ministry of Finance fund for the unemployed, etc.

The Budget transfers to the RHIF a guarantee that, in principle, health insurance coverage is also provided to unemployed, internally-displaced people and refugees, as well as to people who belong to vulnerable categories. A special system of health insurance coverage is applied to the army, army civilians and armed forces' pensioners and their family members and dependents.

Due to the absence of private healthcare insurance, private funding is more or less completely based on out-of-pocket payments and is supplemented by contributions from a small number of major companies which have their own institutions which specialize in the treatment of occupational diseases and also provide primary care services. More than 90% of public costs are financed through the HIF or inter-departmental transfers via the RHIF.

The pharmaceutical market in Serbia in 2013 was approximately € 660.000.000. Serbia's pharmaceutical spending growth will remain depressed for the next two to three years, although all forecasts are optimistic towards the market's long-term growth perspectives.

While the fund is in theory meant to provide universal coverage and reimburse a wide range of services, financial difficulties are prompting the government to raise out-of-pocket expenditure and Serbia's healthcare authorities will continue to cut prices to reduce their pharmaceutical expenditure as a means to contain healthcare costs. In May 2015, the health ministry announced that the prices of around 930 drugs (i.e. drugs related to Alzheimer's and Parkinson's disease, psychosis, depression, osteoporosis, migraine, benign prostatic hyperplasia, bacterial and fungal infections, bronchial asthma, chronic obstructive lung disease, and menopause) are set to become up to 30% cheaper [15].

4.3 Pathways of Market Access (Regulation and Reimbursement)

Albania

In 1994, local authorities had adopted essential drugs list which consisted of 174 products based on the WHO Essential Drugs List mode. Only the pharmaceuticals on this list are reimbursed, either in part or in full, by the Health Insurance Institute (HII). This list is revised from time to time mainly expanding by the introduction of the generics. Drug reimbursement absorbed 70% of the HII budget in 2000 [16].

The public hospitals and ambulatory centers are funded by Ministry of Health, Health insurance institutions, local government, and donations. During 2015 the Ministry of Health (MOH) has announced that it will start the implementation of the project of establishing contemporary costing model and therefore to finance hospital care (grouping based on the diagnosis: Diagnosis Related Groups or DRGs).

Request for introducing new medicines into RL is needed only for including new pharmaceutical dosage forms in the list. If a new drug is registered and its pharmaceutical form dosage is already present in the RL, it is included automatically, ranked according to its price. The requests may come from different sources, but there are the therapeutical committees at the departments of the University Hospital "Mother Theresa" who are responsible for proposing the drugs to the Commission for Assessing and Revising the List of Reimbursable Drugs.

Commission for Assessing and Revising the List of Reimbursable Drugs is appointed by the Minister of Health and is composed of representatives from Ministry of Health, Fund of Compulsory Healthcare Insurance and the University of Medicine. The Minister of Health is responsible for approving the list proposed by the Commission and drafts the list to the Council of Minister. There is no difference between the process of reimbursement of hospital medicines and primary care medicines. The only difference is that these medicines are published in two different lists: Reimbursed drugs lists (for drugs available in community pharmacies) and List of drugs available in the hospital pharmacies.

Proposals for the list of reimbursed drugs are divided into two groups:

1. Changes in RL for diseases whose treatment is already reimbursed. For this purpose, the proposal must be classified in one of the above groups, i.e.: A1, A2, A3, A4. Proposals of group A1, A2, and A3 need support by relevant scientific evidence (e.g. copy of the articles of the current literature, Albanian or international, national scientific forums conclusions or other information based on the proposal). For proposals of group A4 is needed:
   - Data regarding the efficacy of the proposed drug compared to the existing drug in the RL (e.g. photocopy of current literature articles, Albanian or national scientific forums conclusions or any other data);
   - Information on the side effects of the proposed drug, compared with existing drug in RL (e.g. photocopy of current literature articles, Albanian or national scientific forums conclusions or any other data);
   - Comparison of cost treatment between the proposed drug and the existing drug in RL.

2. Changes in the List of Reimbursed Drugs for the treatment of diseases which are not reimbursed or partially reimbursed. For this purpose, the proposal must be classified in one of the above groups, i.e.: B1 or B2. For proposals B1 and B2 groups it is needed :
   - Frequency / incidence of the disease in our country;
   - Role and therapeutic specifications of the proposed drug for the treatment of the disease;
   - Data regarding dosage form, route of administration, daily dosage, criteria for the initiation or termination of the treatment;
   - Criteria showing achievement of the expected effect;
   - Information about the side effects of the proposed drug;
   - The cost of treatment.

For public hospitals the methodology of purchasing consists of three procedures:

1. The most common is the open procedure, when the value of the contract is above the low value threshold (400.000 ALL ≈ 2,875.74 €), through which any interested supplier can submit his offer. The Contracting Authority publishes the procedure on-line (www.app.gov.al) with a minimum time of publication of 25 days. The Contracting Authority in these kinds of tendering is the Ministry of Health.

2. The small value purchase procedures that are used when the purchases are below the low value threshold (400.000 ALL ≈ 2,875.74 €). In this case, the Evaluation Commission shall obtain at least three indications of prices and shall address the contract to the one who offered the best price. Usually in this kind of procedure the Contracting Authorities are the Public Hospitals and the Ambulatory care centers.

3. Negotiated procedure without a prior notice of a contract notice. This procedure has no time limits and it is strictly used when, for reasons of urgency brought about by causes unforeseeable by the Contracting Authority. The Contracting Authority is only the Ministry of Health

For the new products that are registered during the year, the price can be declared at the Minister of Health in the moment when the Order for Registration is issued. The price will be approved within 30 days. The body responsible for determining the price is the Drug Pricing Committee. This committee is chaired by the General Secretary of the MOH and is composed of one representative of the Pharmaceutical Directory at the MOH; one representative of the Ministry of Finance; one representative of the National Agency of Medicines and Medical Devices, and one representative of Fund of Healthcare Compulsory Insurance.

Kosovo

Still, market access policy and rules are not set, so Ministry of Health create policy in order to approve medicines for public financing, especially in hospitals. Since there is no functional Health Insurance Fund, there is no drug reimbursement policy put in place. For hospital needs, medicines and supplies are bought though tender procedure and paid by the state, but for outpatient care, all medicines are bought out of pocket by patients. In regards to pricing, it is free pricing and there are no any rules about pricing and reimbursement still put in place. It is recommended to physicians to prescribe medicines by International Nonproprietary Name (INN) which could be taken as a beginning of generic preference prescribing as a future trend.

4.4 Mapping and structure of Decision Makers

Albania

The main institution that influences the decision of pricing committee is the Ministry of Health. The methodology of determining the price is developed and approved by the MOH and the head of the committee is a representative of the MOH. The price in external reference countries is taken into considerations. The countries included are: Macedonia, Serbia, Croatia, Italy and Greece. The wholesaler's price is being considered.

The price is determined through an approved declared methodology which states that:
- The price of a generic drug must by 20% lower than the one of the patented drug.
- The price declared in Albania must be lower or equal to the lowest price of:
  - The wholesaler's price of the drug in one of the 5 reference countries;
  - The retail price in the country of origin;
  - The declared price in Albania the precedent year.

Drug manufacturer can submit the information regarding the retail price in the country of origin. Only the reference prices are taken into consideration in determining the price. Other studies regarding cost-effectiveness, risk-benefits, clinical trial, cannot influence on the decision.

The prices are declared once a year (from 1st to 31 October). After the new Decision of Council of Ministers no. 645, dated 01.10.2014 on "Functioning of Drug Pricing Committee" has entered into force, the increase of drug price in comparison with the previous year price, is not allowed.

RL including reimbursed price is published once a year at Ministry of Health official website [17]. The medical community has low influence on the decision for market access but in general professional organizations and key opinion leaders who are experts in a specific field can support reimbursement decision through expert opinions on the medical need for some medicines that can satisfy the unmet medical need. Patients organizations exist and often act through increasing awareness on diseases and treatment option but are not officially included in the decision-making process.

Bosnia and Herzegovina

Each entity in Bosnia and Herzegovina is responsible for healthcare finance, management, organization, and provision on its territory, while Brcko District, as a special administrative unit, runs its own healthcare system. According to the administrative organization, there are therefore 13 ministries of health one for Republika Srpska, one for Brcko District, one for the Federation level and ten cantonal ministries in the Federation of Bosnia and Herzegovina (one for each canton).

In brief, the different organizational structures of each entity plus Brcko District are as follows:

- In Republika Srpska, authority over the health system is centralized, with planning, regulation and management functions held by the Ministry of Health and Social.
- In the Federation of Bosnia and Herzegovina, health system administration is decentralized, with each of the ten cantonal administrations having responsibility for the provision of primary and secondary healthcare through its own ministry. The central Ministry of Health of the Federation of Bosnia and Herzegovina coordinates cantonal health administrations at the Federation level. This feature will have obvious functional repercussions in terms of transaction costs, coordination of decision-making at the entity level, and other matters not faced by Republika Srpska.
- The district of Brcko provides primary and secondary care to its citizens.

The concept of decentralization and recentralization is fundamental to understanding the health system of Bosnia and Herzegovina [18].

Federation of Bosnia and Herzegovina

Healthcare system in Federation of Bosnia and Herzegovina is highly decentralized. There are eleven Ministries of Health; on Federal level and at each Canton level. Federal Ministry of health has no authority over cantonal ministries and according to the law has limited functions mainly in terms of coordination.

Operational functions are based and performed by cantonal ministries. They are responsible for service delivery, revenue/insurance collections, expenditures, policy, planning, etc., and each canton operates its own health insurance fund funding healthcare sector – medicines and services provided at cantonal healthcare institutions which are owned by canton and based on its territory [19].

Main financing source in healthcare are public insurance funds including ten cantonal and one Federal health insurance fund. The role of Federal insurance fund is to control and supervise the 11 compulsory insurance funds. Each cantonal government appoints members to its canton's Health Insurance Institute and managing board.

Federal Solidarity, which was established in January 2002, reduces the duplication of services and enable movement of patients from one location to another to receive needed services where available. This will reduce the fragmentation of services between cantons and along ethnic lines. In practical terms, it means that lower income cantons can now equally benefit from expensive interventions that before Solidarity could not be afforded.

This fund mainly cover costs for expensive therapeutics (oncology, biologicals, HI) and procedures (hemodialysis, transplantation etc.). Federal MoH publishes the list of medicines that can be funded by Solidarity fund and process contains submission of reimbursement dossier including pharmacoeconomics analysis (mainly budget impact and cost-effectiveness) with local data [20].

After the list is adopted, Fund announces a tender for purchase medicines included into the list. Criteria for selection are that lowest offered price/supplier is accepted. This tender is announced each year after the list has been revised.

Law on Health Insurance from 1997 defined that insurance is "obligatory in the territory of the Canton". Health insurance contributions are paid by employees and their family members are subsequently insured. Contribution rates and methods of calculating and paying contributions for compulsory health insurance are determined by the Federal Ministry of Finance. Cantonal health insurance funds can determine their own rates but they cannot exceed or must be equal to those established by the Federal Ministry of Finance and Law on Contributions. The current average contribution rate of 18% of salary consists of 13% paid for by the employee and 5% by the employer.

Cantons annually submit a compulsory insurance scheme plans to its cantonal minister for the approval. In case that expenditures exceed the planned incomes, the cantonal budget could cover this gap.

Each of ten cantonal funds then administers their money and allocate resources to the providers. Cantons may also autonomously introduce the so-called "extended health insurance" in order to extend coverage for services not covered under the entity's compulsory health insurance system [18].

In order to establish unified access to medicines, Federal MoH put in place Ordinance on criteria for medicines introduction into the list. The general concept is that in Federation there are 2 reimbursement lists. List A which is obligatory to all cantonal Health Insurance Fund (HIF) and price set on the list during the negotiation process with MoH must be paid 100% by cantonal HIF. List B consists of medicines that are recommended for reimbursement at cantonal level with different copayment level. This depends on cantonal budgets, and the list can be decreased or expanded with additional drugs depending on cantonal funds.

Each year Federal list is revised causing price decrease of drugs included into the list (on average 10%). Submission and introduction of new medicines require pharmacoeconomic part reimbursement dossier including budget impact analysis and cost-effectiveness analysis [19].

Republika Srpska

Republika Srpska Ministry of Health and Social Welfare is centralized with regard to administrative, regulatory and fiscal responsibilities.

Health Insurance Fund of the Republic of Srpska is the only body responsible for collection and allocation of financial contributions and this fund operates on the basis of solidarity and mutuality. Republika Srpska's Health Insurance Fund consists of 8 regional offices and 54 branch offices with a high level of centralization. Regional offices are, however, partly autonomous, since they operate with around 80% of the income collected in the territory they cover; on the other hand, branch offices have no autonomy in decision-making. The central office of this Fund is responsible for the overall strategy and operations. It sets prices of services and goods paid by the fund.

According to the 1999 Law on Health Insurance, compulsory social health insurance is expected to provide coverage for insured people, their family members, and members of their household.

As supplementary funding out-of-pocket and different co-payment schemes has been introduced in order to cover budget gaps and ensure sustainability of the fund. Opt-in or voluntary insurance is not introduced and recognized, but so-called extended insurance has been introduced. It is supplementary insurance with extra benefits, including the risk of co-payments [18].

In the Republic of Srpska HIF publishes three reimbursement lists: List A with 100% reimbursement, list B with 50% co-payment, and a list of hospital and cytotoxic drugs. Hospital and cytotoxic drugs are purchased through tenders (lowest offered price/supplier win tender and provide supply for 2 years) [21]. Revision of reimbursement list for primary healthcare is performed on annual basis.

Macedonia, FYR

Pharmaceutical sector, as well as the whole healthcare system, has passed through different reforms in the Republic of Macedonia in recent years. One of the most achievements in this reform process was the establishment and implementation of "Methodology on the manner of establishment of medication prices" which was introduced in 2011 [22]. This methodology is related to the establishment of the wholesale and retail prices of prescription drugs that have obtained Marketing Authorization. In its basics it is referral pricing system based on prices in the following referral countries: Republic of Slovenia, Republic of Bulgaria, the Netherlands, Republic of Poland, the United Kingdom, Republic of France, Republic of Croatia, Republic of Serbia, Republic of Greece, Federal Republic of Germany, Republic of Turkey and the Russian Federation. This act prices of drugs has been significantly reduced and other activities such regulation of generic medicines promotion resulted in significant increase in the number of reimbursable drugs on the positive list. In 2013, the Health Insurance Fund implemented reimbursement list consisted of 391 generic drugs that are included in the positive list, 299 are provided at no additional charge. In comparison to the positive (reimbursement) list from 2009, a number of reimbursed drugs has been significantly increased, especially with drugs with no additional charge or co-payment. Price control has also contributed to significant savings to healthcare budgets and available funds.

From 2012 two Positive lists for drugs had been introduced: List A which include drugs for primary healthcare and list B which include drugs for hospital healthcare.

The reimbursement criteria are:

- Price of drugs based on DDD;
- Total cost of treatment per patient;
- Total cost for one year treatment for chronic therapy;
- Cost-minimization analysis for the same indication;
- Comparative efficacy (cost/effects) with other drugs for the same indication;
- Expected number of patients and budget impact;
- Countries in which candidate drug is on list of reimbursement drugs;
- Drug therapeutically committees – Committees for "positive list".

All hospital medicines are being purchased through tendering and are oriented towards medicines included in referral list for hospital medicines (e-auctions). Each public hospital must plan annual tenders in their annual budget which is approved by Ministry of health. Public hospitals usually pay the suppliers which were selected during tenders, in the period from 6 months to 2 years, after delivery of medicines.

It is important to notice that Macedonian market is specific because parallel import is authorized and this is one of government measures to reduce pharmaceutical expenditure, especially for expensive drugs. Law on medicines allows a parallel trade for medicines with market authorization in the EU, Switzerland, Norway, Canada, Japan, Israel and USA, and has market authorization in Macedonia as well. Agency for medicines approves a parallel trade to wholesalers who obtain required documents.

Montenegro

There is just public health financing and specificity in Montenegro in comparison to other countries is that all pharmaceuticals included into HIF reimbursement list are purchased through central tender. There is no co-payment, but drugs that are not reimbursed are purchased by pocket money and level of out-of-pocket sales is not officially measured.

Even there are no clear criteria established in regards to the introduction of new medicines to reimbursement list, Health insurance fund establishing prices of medicines using some criteria like the average price of the product in referral countries (Slovenia, Serbia, and Croatia) and pharmacoeconomics criteria but now specified which exactly. This calculation of average referral price defines maximal prices, but the price on tender can be lower and this price is reimbursed.

Serbia

Pharmaceutical pricing is under the following mechanism: MoH and Ministry of trade jointly define maximal market price based on the average of three referent countries and defined artificial exchange rate (usually below official rate) published in Price Decree. Reimbursement price is regulated by Insurance fund and price is the minimum of 3 referent countries (Slovenia, Croatia, and Italy).

From 2013, centralized procurement system has been introduced with the main intention to improve the difficult situation in public healthcare system. This is also one of the most important anti-corruption measures. It is estimated that 20%-50% savings will be made through this procurement system mainly due to pharmaceutical price decrease especially in the case of high-volume products. This system has been extended from public pharmacies to private pharmacies too [23].

Drug reimbursed by National HIF are those included in 4 types of reimbursement list marked as A, A1, B and C. Products included in list A and A1 are mainly used in primary care, while list B and C include products used in the hospital setting.

Application to reimbursement list is evaluated by NHIF and required documentation are basic pharmacoeconomic analysis CEA/CUA/BIM for innovative, and CMA for generics at the insurance Fund. Positive opinion needed for reimbursement decision, by PE Committee at the Fund. One chapter of reimbursement file is the mandatory section to submit. PE committee only formally confirms negotiation decisions and approves agreements. It is It is possible to sign the special agreement, both financial or outcome based on shared risk.

.5 Challenges and catalyzers for Market Access and Look-up for Near Future

Albania

It can be expected that the future trends will be focused on additional savings due to budget restrictions and generic penetration. It is also expected that official market access rules will be implemented in order to increase transparency but also access to novel therapies. Access to EU will surely improve this processes.

Bosnia and Herzegovina

Due to highly decentralization healthcare system efficacy is very low; at the same time, market access is slow due to multiple parallel processes that reimbursement applicant must pass. The budget investment could be improved through centralization of decision making and resources allocation, especially in Federation of Bosnia and Herzegovina where we face with multiple health insurance funds (10 cantonal and Federal HIF). Due to budget restrictions, the current trend is price pressure while saved money is not allocated to novel therapies but other healthcare costs like salaries and hospital programs. EU integration process could have a positive impact on the full implementation of HTA and decision-making. The current legislation made the good framework and create good predispositions for implementation of HTA but the development of this area will include capacity building and mainly political decisions for further improvements.

Kosovo

It is expected that the recently created Health insurance fund will establish market access rules and make the process more transparent. The main catalyzer would be EU access process through legislation adoption.

Macedonia, FYR

The current trend of price pressure seems to be unsustainable due to the risk of withdrawal of some manufacturers. Even market access process is established through regulation pricing block introduction of new molecules into reimbursement system. Also, parallel trade which allows additionally complicate this situation. If this trend continues it could be expected that most of the funding could be private or pocket money thorough copayments or full payments by the patients.

As it is the case in all Western Balkan countries, Macedonia also faces with the lack of experts in the field of HTA and pharmacoeconomics/health economics. Some non-government professional associations implemented non-academic education in this field and work on awareness increase for the necessity of this processes in order to improve the decision-making process.

Montenegro

It is expected that the future trend will be the introduction of the private sector into the system and further price decreases.

Serbia

The Serbian pharmaceutical market, as the biggest in the region, is very important and impact trends in neighboring countries and region. Price pressure and policies have a direct impact on prices in countries where Serbia is one of the references. It is expected that HTA will continue development in the near future. There are possibilities to create risk sharing agreements, especially for innovative products, and this could be huge opportunity not just in Serbia but also the region in order to assure better access to novel therapies.

4.6 **References**

1. Timeline: Break-up of Yugoslavia. BBC News. Available at http://news.bbc.co.uk/2/hi/europe/4997380.stm (last accessed June 2016)
2. The International Criminal Tribunal for the former Yugoslavia (ICTY).Available at http://www.icty.org/sid/321 (last accessed July 2015)

3. Grielen SJ, Boerma WG, Groenwegen PP. Unity of diversity? Task profiles of general Practitioners in Central and Eastern Europe. *Eur J Public* Health 2000; 10: 249-54
4. Bredenkamp C, Gragnolati M. Sustainability of Healthcare Financing in the Western Balkans: An Overview of Progress and Challenges. The World Bank Europe and Central Asia Region Human Development Department. 2007
5. Souliotis K, Economou C, Tountas Y. Health Care Reforms in the Ex-Socialist South-Eastern European Countries. *Journal of Societal & Social Policy* 2005; 4: 63-76
6. The World Bank Data. Available at http://data.worldbank.org/ (last accessed August 2015)
7. Imasheva A, Seiter A. HNP Discussion Paper – The Pharmaceutical Sector of the Western Balkan Countries. The World Bank. 2008.
8. Nuri B. In: Tragakes E (ed.). Heath care systems in transition: Albania. Copenhagen: European Observatory on Health Care Systems, 2002
9. Ministry of Civil Affairs of Bosnia and Herzegovina. Available at http://www.mcp. gov.ba (last accessed May 2015)
10. Agency for medicines and medical devices of Bosnia and Herzegovina. Available at http://www.almbih.gov.ba/ (last accessed May 2015)
11. Health Policy Institute (HPI). Available at http://www.hpi.sk/en/2013/11/ kosovobrief-health-system-review/ (last accessed August 2015)
12. Health Insurance Fund of Montenegro. Available at http://fzocg.me (last accessed July 2015)
13. Health Care system and financing in Serbia. Available at http://ceves.org.rs/ wpcontent/uploads/2014/01/Health-Care-System-and-Spending-in-Serbia.pdf (last accessed July 2015)
14. Health Policy Institute (HPI). Health care system in Serbia. Available at http://www.hpi.sk/en/2014/01/serbia-brief-health-system-review/ (last accessed July 2015)
15. BMI Research. Serbia Pharmaceuticals & Healthcare Report. Available at http://store.bmiresearch.com/serbia-pharmaceuticals-healthcare-report.html (last accessed: August 2015)
16. International Monetary Fund. Albania. Growth and poverty reduction strategy 2001-2004
17. Ministry of Health of Albania. Reimbursement list. Available at http://www.shendetesia.gov.al/al/publikime/farmaceutika/dokumenta-te-publikuara-ngadrejtoria-farmaceutike-ne-vitet-2008-2014 (last accessed August 2015)
18. Cain J. In Cain J, Jakubowski, E (eds). Heath care systems in transition: Bosnia and Herzegovina. Copenhagen: European Observatory on Health Care Systems, 2002
19. Federal Ministry of Health. Available at http://www.fmoh.gov.ba/ (last accessed May 2015)
20. Federal Health Insurance Fund. Available at http://www.fedzzo.com.ba/bs/clanak/ fond-solidarnosti/38 (last accessed September 2016)

21. Health Insurance Fund of Republic of Srpska. Available at http://www.zdravstvosrpske.org/ (last accessed May 2015)
22. Dauti M, Alili-Idrizi E, Ahmeti-Lika S. Overview on generic policies and pharmaceutical pricing in the European countries and The Republic of Macedonia. *European Scientific Journal* 2015; 11: 302-8
23. HIS Markit. Serbian government intervenes to save pharmaceutical market and announces launch of centralised public procurement for healthcare. Available at https://www.ihs.com/country-industry-forecasting.html?ID=1065973831 (last accessed August 2015)

Market Access in North Eastern Europe Countries

Esin Tuna
With the collaboration of Marina Lesnicheva, Pawel Mierzejewski and Olexandr Topachevskyi

General Outlook of Healthcare System and Health Policies

Russia

The Russian healthcare system's infrastructure is inherited from the Soviet Union. The system is highly centralized and focused on universal access to basic care despite the evolution over the past 20 years.

The dominant institutions in the Russian health system are the Ministry of Health (MoH) and Social Development (MoHSD), with its associated federal services *Rospotrebnadzor, Roszdravnadzor*, the Federal Medical and Biological Agency (FMBA), and the Federal Mandatory Health Insurance (MHI) Fund. Each level in the state organizational hierarchy reports to the state body directly superior to it (Figure 1).

In each region, the gubernatorial administration has a health department that oversees regionally owned health facilities (multipurpose and specialized hospitals, specialized clinics, outpatient facilities, diagnostic centers, specialized emergency care facilities, etc.) and monitors municipal-level health departments and their respective facilities. Municipalities oversee those health facilities they own. In urban municipalities, the medical facility network comprises general and specialized hospitals, polyclinics, emergency care facilities, diagnostic centers, and so on. The network in rural municipalities usually consists of general hospitals (the central rayon hospital), rayon hospitals and small village (*uchastkovye*) hospitals. Primary care in rural facilities is provided by the outpatient departments of rural hospitals and feldsher-midwife posts (Feldshersko-Akusherskiy Punkt – FAP), which are usually supervised by the nearest rural hospital. In addition to the hierarchy and assets of the MoHSD, several ministries continue to operate "parallel" health systems of ministerial polyclinics, hospitals, sanatoria and public health facilities [1].

The socialist model of healthcare providing free healthcare for all citizens, before 1990s, was collapsed due to the insufficiency of investment and infrastructure [2]. In 2005, Russian government launched National Priority Project (NPP). The NPP Program was aimed at developing social welfare in Russia by 4 selected projects focusing on public health, education, housing and agriculture. In this regard, the healthcare sector had re-

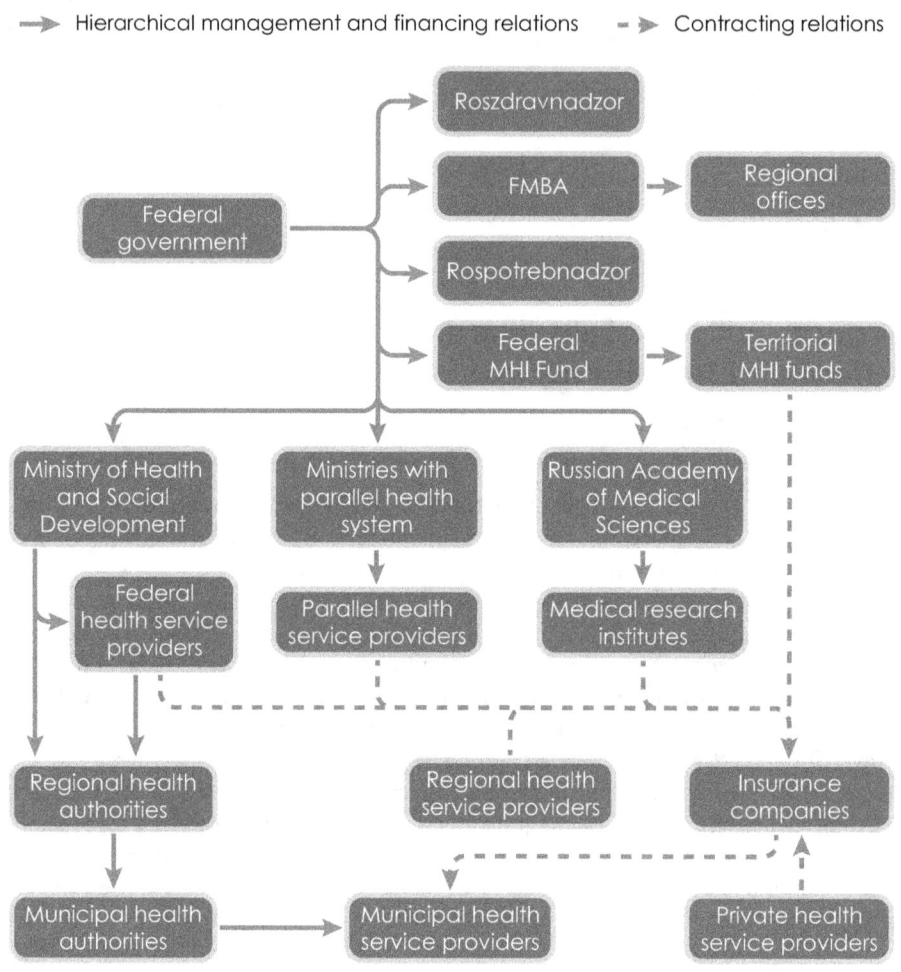

Figure 1. Overview of Russian healthcare system. Modified from [1]
FMBA = Federal Medical and Biological Agency; MHI = Mandatory Health Insurance

ceived significant funding that it has never received for several decades [3]. Named as The National Priority Project on Health 2007-2012, its main objectives included extension of life expectancy in general, lowering the infant mortality rate and improvement of preventive outpatient primary care [4].

The current healthcare system in Russia is based on budget and insurance model of funding that involves state and regionally owned medical organizations, which is being managed by the Russian MoH. The Russian healthcare system mainly bases on the annually adopted Program of State Guarantees of Free Medical Treatment to Russian Citizens (the "State Program") in which the types and conditions of medical treatment, standards of scope of medical aid, standards of financial expenses per specific item of medical aid, per capita standards of financial expenses, formation procedure and structure of tariffs of medical aid are defined. It also provides criteria of quality and accessibility of medical aid provided free of charge to the citizens of Russia within its territory [5].

The State Program for 2014 was adopted by the Russian Government's Resolution No. 932 dated 18 October 2013 "On Program of State Guarantees of Free Medical Treatment to the Citizens for 2014 and Planned Period of 2015 and 2016". According to the State Program for 2014 the following is guaranteed for the citizens for free [6]:

- Primary medical aid;
- Specialized medical aid (including, high-tech medical aid provided in accordance with list of such aid adopted by the Russian MoH;
- Emergency medical aid (including specialized);
- Palliative medical aid.

Medical insurance in Russia is composed of mandatory medical insurance (OMS), which is being provided under the State program and voluntary medical insurance (DMS) [5].

OMS is covers the following principles:

- Universal coverage, which means the equality of right for obtaining medical aid despite age, gender, status, state of health;
- Governmental coverage which means the state provides rational use of OMS funds and fulfillment of its obligations before insured individuals;
- Non-commercial coverage, which means all sums are addressed for the system of OMS and medical institutions.

OMS guarantees Russian citizens the right to obtain free of charge medical and pharmaceutical aid within the scope of particular programs of OMS. OMS covers primary medical aid, specialized medical aid (excluding high-tech medical aid), and the list of relevant medical aid and supply of medicines in case of particular diseases (the list as integral part of the OMS may be altered from year to year The medicines are provided to in-hospital patients, others need to purchase medicines out of pocket. Hospital care is provided in accordance with Essential Drugs List, which is reviewed once a year and National Standards of treatment).

DMS system is supplementary to the OMS, provides greater coverage in terms of medical services, but needs to be separately purchased. For the moment, the employers usually purchase this type of insurance as an additional benefit for the employees.

Poland

The Polish healthcare system was strictly hierarchical and predominantly funded from the central budget before the start of gradual public sector devolution in 1989. The strongly centralized system based on the Soviet model of healthcare (the so-called Semashko model) was replaced with a decentralized system of mandatory health insurance, comple-

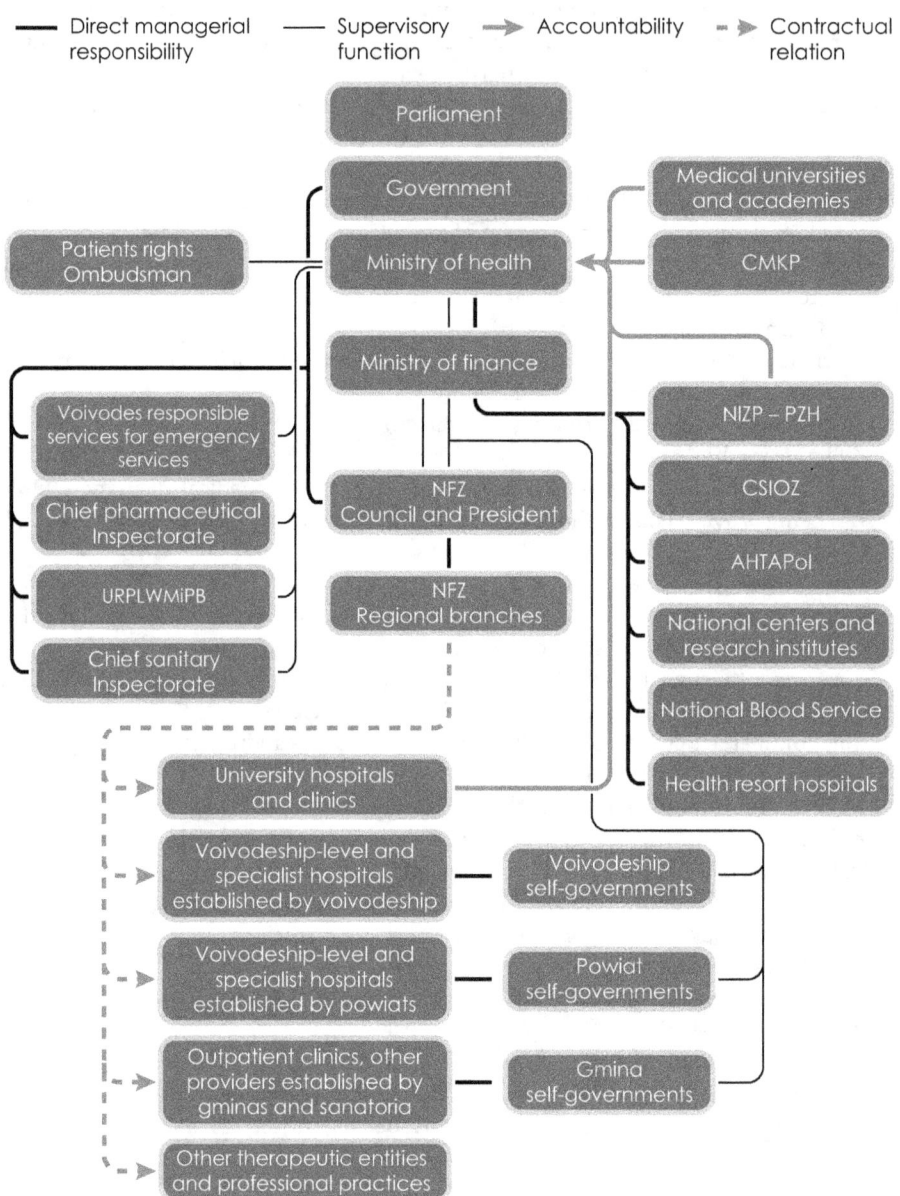

Figure 2. Overview of the structure of the Polish health system [7]

AHTAPol = National Agency for Health Technology Assessment and Tarification; CSIOZ = Center for Health Information Systems; NFZ = National Health Fund; CMKP = Medical Center of Postgraduate Education; NIZP = National Institute of Public Health; PZH = National Institute of Hygiene; URPLWMiPB = Office for the registration of pharmaceuticals, Medical Devices and Biocides mented with financing from central and local budgets during the political and economic reorganization that followed the collapse of communism. In this regard, the administration of most healthcare services and the ownership of most public healthcare facilities were transferred to *voivodeships* and *gminas* (municipality) and later also to *powiats* (districts) from MoH, during 1990s.

The main bodies responsible for the management and finance of the Polish healthcare system are the MoH, the National Health Fund (NFZ) and territorial self-governments. NFZ is primarily responsible for funding of healthcare services for insured population and managing the contracting process with public and non-public and private service providers under the supervision of MoH. At national level, MoH is primarily responsible for national health policy, finance of long term public health programs, several highly specialized medical services, major capital investments and medical education. At each administrative level, territorial health authorities (*gmina, powiat, voivodeship*) are responsible for assessment of the adequacy of service provision and healthcare infrastructure, determination of health needs, planning of health services delivery, health promotion and prevention and the management of public health institutions. A simplified overview of the structure of the Polish health system is given in Figure 2.

All citizens, regardless of their financial status, have the right to equally access to health services that are financed from public funds. The compulsory health insurance system covers approximately 98% of the population including the family members of persons contributing to the insurance and some vulnerable groups whose contributions are financed from the state budget. Membership in social health insurance scheme is mandatory for the vast majority of the citizens and legal residents. The population without health insurance coverage through NFZ is still allowed to receive free healthcare services at the point of delivery.

NFZ provides a very broad range of healthcare services including:
- Primary healthcare (internal medicine, emergency medicine, family medicine);
- Ambulatory specialist care;
- Hospital treatment;
- Psychiatric care and addiction treatment;
- Therapeutic rehabilitation;
- Nursing and long-term care services;
- Dental treatment;
- Health resort treatment;
- Provision of orthopedic and auxiliary medical devices;
- Medical rescue services;
- Palliative and hospice care;
- Highly specialized services (e.g. transplant surgery);
- Health programs;
- Pharmaceuticals;

There are no differences between insured groups in terms of guaranteed scope of services except reimbursement of pharmaceuticals and auxiliary pharmaceutical appliances [7].

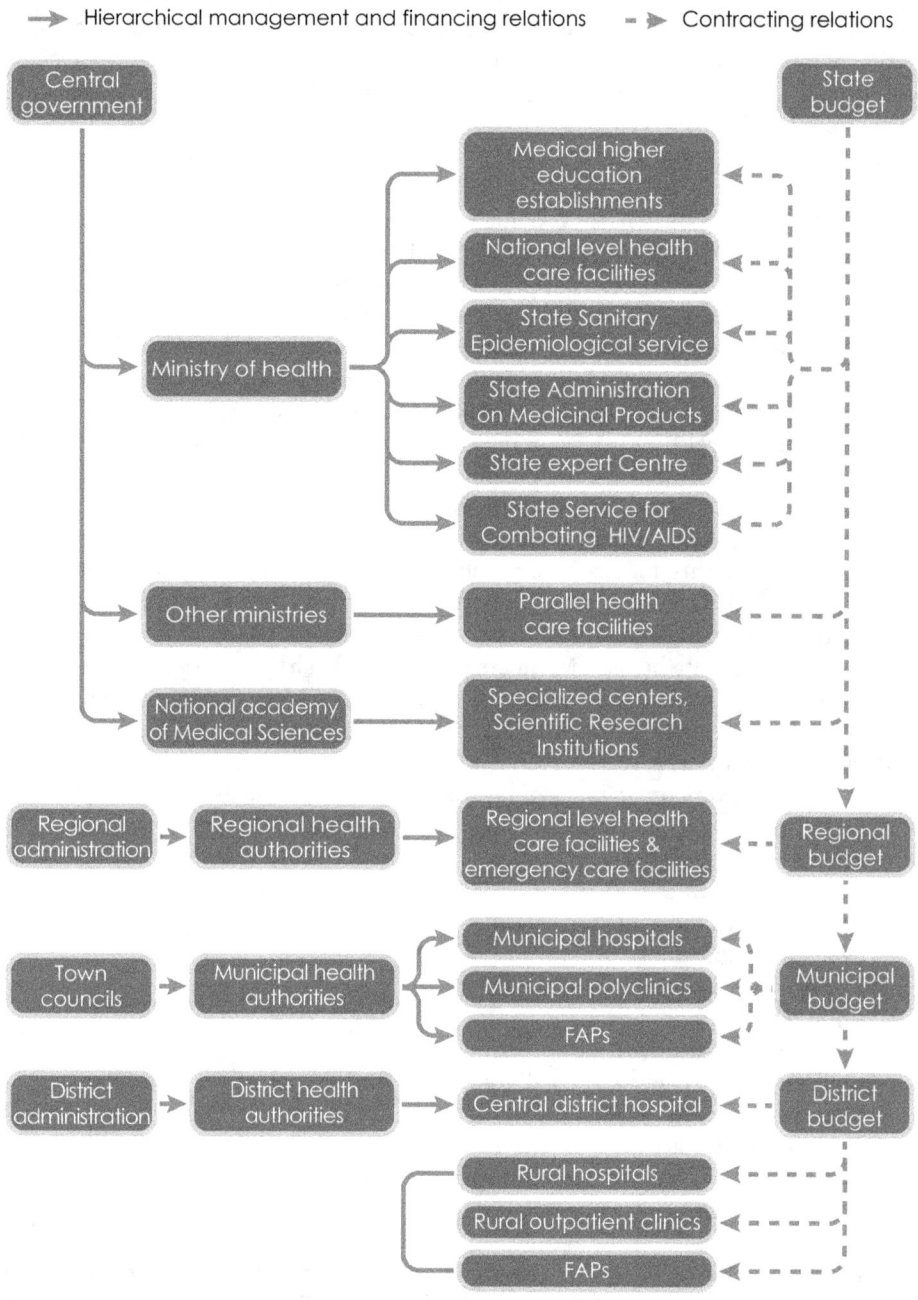

Figure 3. Overview of the Ukrainian health system [8]

Ukraine

The Ukrainian healthcare system is based on Semashko system, which was adopted in 1991 and couldn't be sustained due to the economic downturn confronted after independence. After independence, not being so ultimate, some changes have been promoted and actualized in the healthcare sector. In this regard, the latest reform package, consisting of three phases to be implemented in a four-year period (2010-2014) was introduced to be valid from 2010. Primarily in phase one, changes in healthcare financing were targeted in order to reduce fragmentation and prioritize primary care. Secondarily, a pilot program was aimed to be implemented in four regions consisting of Donetsk, Dnipropetrovsk, Vinnytsya oblasts and Kyiv city. Thirdly, it was aimed to expand those reforms, however these plans are postponed due to the unstable political situation [8].

The system is officially designed to be financed through general taxation and ensure universal access to unlimited care, which is provided free at public healthcare facilities. However, patients usually need to pay out of pocket to access services in practice [8].

The main statutory system is coordinated and governed by the Ministry of Health and the parallel systems are governed trough their respective ministries. At regional level, the regional health authorities are responsible for implementation of national health policies within their territory and management of regional healthcare facilities primarily providing specialized and highly specialized services as well as emergency care services. At regions, districts or municipal levels, most of the healthcare services are provided through these facilities under local government and financed through the budget of relevant body of the government that receives the budget from the relative government level (Figure 3). Nevertheless, patients may require paying for outpatient and inpatient pharmaceuticals due to the insufficient government financing [8].

All Ukrainian citizens are covered by a comprehensive guaranteed package of healthcare services provided free of charge at the point of use due to the Article 49 of the Constitution of Ukraine of 1996. However, this expansive universal coverage couldn't be supported by adequate financing. Therefore, government inclined to limit the guaranteed package of free healthcare. In 2002, the government approved a new list of healthcare services that could be provided for a fee, to be fully paid by the patient or a third party at state healthcare facilities. In 2002 government also approved the Program for Providing the Citizens of Ukraine with Free Health Care Guaranteed by the state giving a defined list of healthcare services could be provided free at state health care facilities. The program includes:

- Emergency care:
- Outpatient polyclinic care:
- Inpatient care for acute conditions and emergencies requiring intensive treatment; 24 hour medical surveillance and hospitalization:
- Emergency dental care and comprehensive care for children, disabled people, students, pregnant women and women with children under 3 years of age:
- First aid for rural population:
- Specialized care for disabled people and children:
- Medical care for children in orphanages.

The proportion of the population covered by voluntary health insurance varies between 2.4% and 3.3% of the overall population in 2013 due to article written by Lekhan in 2014 [8]. The market share of voluntary health insurance has remained at about 0.9% of the total health expenditures. It has two main roles as complementary and supplementary. As being complementary, it covers payments for pharmaceuticals and access to different services that could not financed by the statuary health insurance. As being supplementary, it provides greater choice of provider by ensuring its patients to access most exclusive facilities and higher level of comfort and faster access to healthcare services [8].

5.2 Pathways of Market Access

Russia

Pricing of pharmaceuticals

The price of pharmaceuticals takes part in the list of essential and most important pharmaceuticals (Essential Drug List), which is regulated and controlled by the state. The principles of the state regulation on pharmaceutical pricing are defined in the Law on Circulation of Medicines and Government Resolution "On the State Regulation of Prices of Medicines Included into the List of Essential and Most Important Medicines" No. 865 dated 15 August 2015 ("Resolution 979") [6].

The pharmaceuticals are specified by their international non-proprietary name (INN) and pharmaceutical form in the Essential Drug List. The Essential Drug List is updated once a year [6].

The prices of the pharmaceuticals included into the Essential Drug List are influenced by two principles.

- The registration of maximum manufacturer's prices of pharmaceuticals by the state. This price is calculated due to the government's approach that gives an estimation of (i) average actual selling price, (ii) average actual importation price, and (iii) expenses for development, production and sale of medicines, indication of the minimum manufacturer's prices in the manufacturer's state and other states, where the medicine is registered, taking into account expenses for customs clearance and transportation. The maximum manufacturer's price is estimated due to the following principles:
- Referring to Russian manufacturers – the price of analogue pharmaceutical agents produced on the territory of the Russian federation corresponding with their INN, dosage form and dosing. If such an analogues is not available, the price of foreign analogues that are in circulation in the territory of the Russian Federation;
- Referring to foreign manufacturers – the price of analogue pharmaceutical agents that circulates in the civil territory of the Russian Federation corresponding with their INN, dosage form and dosing.

The maximum manufacturer's prices of pharmaceuticals, which are registered properly and included into the Essential Drug List, are indicated in the related state register.

The pharmaceuticals that are included into the Essential Drug list are prohibited to be imported and circulate in the Russian market until and unless their maximum manufacturer's price is registered according to the above mentioned principles.

- The determination of maximum wholesale and retail trade margins applied to prices of pharmaceuticals which is affected at the regional level. Under the Law on Circulation of Medicines, the maximum wholesale and retail trade margins for pharmaceuticals included in the Essential Drug List are determined by regional governmental authorities corresponding to the approach approved by the Government of the Russian Federation. Wholesalers and/or pharmacy organizations, individual entrepreneurs having a pharmaceutical activity license shall sell pharmaceuticals included into the Essential Drug List at prices not exceeding the actual manufacturer's selling price (which shall not exceed the registered maximum manufacturer's price) and the amount of respective wholesale and retail trade margins determined by regional governmental authorities. Prices for other pharmaceuticals, which are not included into the Essential Drug List, and medical devices, are not regulated by the state.

There is no initial price negotiation for a newly launched pharmaceutical. The price level of a medicinal preparation may in certain circumstances depend on the prices for the same product in other countries.

Reimbursement of Pharmaceuticals

There is no such a reimbursement system as exists in European countries. According to the current legislation, inpatient pharmaceuticals are covered for free and outpatient pharmaceuticals are paid for in full out of pocket. Nonetheless there are several governmental programs that provide pharmaceuticals for free or with 50% discount to patients that have certain diseases and or belonging to certain categories of citizens (social security beneficiaries) [9]. The groups of citizens eligible for such benefits are determined by the federal authorities, although regional authorities can, in addition, provide benefits for other groups [1].

Outpatient pharmaceuticals are financed through several different public sources such as the federal budget, regional budgets and compulsory health insurance (Figure 2) [10].

For patients meeting the criteria stated below, the federal budget fully reimburses outpatient pharmaceuticals.

- **The ONLS program.** Patients under this scheme have the right to receive "a set of social services" including fully reimbursed outpatient pharmaceuticals. The patient groups eligible for this program includes veterans of wars, Leningrad siege medalholders, others who worked on specific objectives during World War II, family members of those killed or disabled in action, disabled individuals, and disabled children. The list of pharmaceuticals provided under this program is determined by MoH.
- **The VZN program.** Also known as "Seven Nosologies" program, this program ensures patients to receive high-cost pharmaceuticals related to several diseases like hemophilia, mucoviscidosis, multiple sclerosis and Gaucher's disease. The list of pharmaceuticals provided under this program is determined by the government.

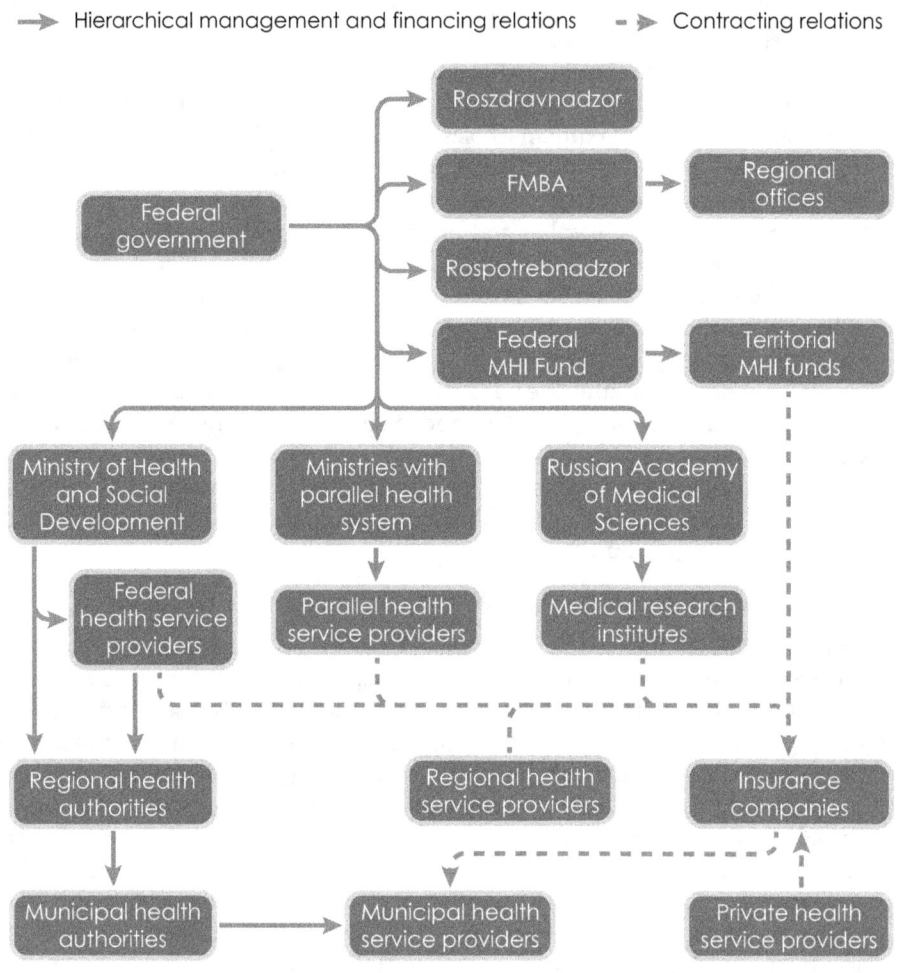

Figure 2. Pharmaceuticals Provision in Russia by Source of Financing. Modified from [1,10]
FFOMS = Federal Fund for Mandatory Medical Insurance

- **Other**. Pharmaceuticals for patients that have dangerous infectious diseases such as HIV/AIDS, tuberculosis etc., are covered at federal level. The list of pharmaceuticals provided under this program is determined by federal government.

The ONLS and VZN program are referred as the Dopolnitel'noe Lekarstevennoe Obespechenie (DLO) scheme.

For patients meeting the criteria stated below, the territorial and regional governments are theoretically required to fund outpatient pharmaceuticals.

- **Patients suffering from orphan diseases.** There is no specific list of pharmaceuticals reimbursed under this program.
- **Certain other groups.** Children under three years of age, people exposed to radiation as a result of the Chernobyl nuclear power plant disaster, or as a result of nuclear testing at the Semipalatinsk range, and patients suffering from certain diseases (e.g. diabetes mellitus and cancer) are included in these groups. The list of pharmaceuticals provided under for these groups is determined by regional authorities. As there is lack of certainty of regulations defined by the guidelines, there may be huge differences between regions in terms of level provision of healthcare services.

Pharmaceuticals, provided in inpatient and emergency care units, are reimbursed via compulsory health insurance under the Federal Fund for Mandatory Medical Insurance (FFOMS). Besides the fact that the patients are guaranteed to receive free of charge medical aid including the pharmaceuticals listed in the Essential Drug List in hospital settings, they may also receive some pharmaceuticals that are not included into the Essential Drug List due to the vital indications or other several reasons [5].

Besides all that stated above, Russian healthcare legislation does not cover the off-label use and regulates the supply of medicines in accordance with their approved indications.

Poland

Pricing of Pharmaceuticals

Assessment of quality, efficacy and safety of pharmaceuticals, medical devices and biocidal products are under the responsibilities of The Office for Registration of Pharmaceuticals, Medical Devices and Biocidal Products (URPLWMiPB) which is a governmental agency directly subordinated to the Minister of Health. President of the URPLWMiPB control the safety of pharmaceuticals and discloses the market authorizations and have the right to withdraw a previously granted market authorization in case of an unexpected, severe or life-threatening adverse effects or lack of declared therapeutic efficacy.

Pharmaceuticals can be registered through three procedures all-compliant with EU standards: centralized, decentralized and mutual recognition. Authorized pharmaceuticals are registered by the President of the URPLWMiPB. Market authorizations are valid for five years and if requested by market authorization holder, they can be extended [7].

Price controls effects reimbursed products only and these products' official selling price including VAT is determined by the reimbursement decision. Reimbursed products are tributary to price controls and their official wholesale margins (5% of the official selling price) and retail margins (according to amount/percentage rates determined by law) are determined in the law. Both the official selling prices and official wholesale and retail margins are fixed for outpatient pharmaceuticals. Prices and margins for inpatients treatment have maximal character. Prices and margins for products without reimbursement decisions may be determined freely by their manufacturers.

An official selling price is determined by reimbursement decision. The Minister of Health sets the official selling price taking into consideration:

- Position of the Economic Commission (a body established by the Minister of Health within the official reimbursement process);
- Recommendation of the President of AHTAPol, with special emphasis on the analysis of the relation between the incurred costs and the achieved health effects (EBM and HTA based);
- Price competitiveness.

The official selling price for outpatient pharmacies market is the basis for calculation of a fixed wholesale margin amounting to five percent, and then a fixed retail margin according to percentage/amount rates specified by law.

The price for a given reimbursed product to be paid by the patient is, therefore, the same at every pharmacy and equals the official selling price specified by reimbursement decision, plus the wholesale and retail margin [5].

Reimbursement of Pharmaceuticals

Pharmaceuticals are reimbursed if they are authorized for marketing and are marketed (with an exception for named-patient basis import), if they are available on the market and if they have an EAN (International Article Number) or another unique code equivalent to EAN.

Unlike the these pharmaceuticals, the following may not be reimbursed:
- A pharmaceutical in clinical conditions in which it is possible to effectively replace such a product by changing the patient's lifestyle;
- Prescription pharmaceutical, which has an OTC counterpart, unless it requires administration for more than 30 days in a specific clinical condition;
- Pharmaceutical obtained by way of named-patient basis import, specified in an applicable ordinance of the Minister of Health.

The Law on the Reimbursement of Drugs, Food for Special Medical Purposes (FSMPs) and Medical Devices from 2011 from 2011 provides for the following reimbursement availability category:
- Available in the pharmacy on the prescription (within the whole scope of registered indications and intended uses or for indications specified by a given clinical condition);
- Used within the scope of a pharmaceutical program;
- Used in chemotherapy (within the whole scope of registered indications and intended uses or for indications specified by a given clinical condition);
- Used within the scope of providing guaranteed services other than the above-listed.

Ministry of Health is the decision maker entity in the reimbursement of a pharmaceutical and the Economic Committee, the AHTAPol and the Transparency Council are the other entities officially involved in the reimbursement procedure.

Not exceeding the market exclusivity period, a validity period of the reimbursement decision may be issued for five, three or two years. After the termination of the reimbursement decision, a new reimbursement motion has to be filed to the Minister of Health [5].

According to the law from 2011 reimbursed pharmaceuticals are available to all insured persons:

- Free of charge (pharmaceutical proven to be effective in cancer treatment, some psychiatric conditions or severe infectious diseases);
- At a fixed fee (for pharmaceuticals on the basic drugs list defined in the 2011 and for pharmaceuticals normally requiring a 30% or 50% co-payment when therapy lasts longer than 30 days and the monthly cost of treatment exceeds 5% or 30% of the minimum wage, respectively);
- For 50% of the price (for therapies shorter than 30 days);
- For 30% of the price in other cases.

The Ministry of Health decides whether cost-sharing to be applied on pharmaceuticals and medical devices reimbursement and defines the extent on the official sales price and confidential risk-sharing instruments (if applicable). The decision is issued for five, three or two years. First and second decision for the product has to be given for two years and next would be longer. In making reimbursement decisions, the Ministry of Health is supported by AHTAPol as the main reimbursement advisor issued by the Reimbursement Law and the Economic Commission (the official body established by the MoH for negotiation of price and final reimbursement conditions process. The final MoH decision is based on the President of AHTAPol recommendation and the opinion of the Economic Commission. In decision-making process are taken into account: clinical, cost-effectiveness and safety profiles of the pharmaceutical, as well as its health benefits and budget impact; the availability of clinical alternatives; and existing health priorities [7].

The lists of reimbursed drugs and medical devices are published by the Ministry and updated every two months.

Despite, the National Pharmaceutical Policy for 2004-2008 identified a need for the development of ambulatory healthcare formularies, which would contain guidelines on the use of pharmaceuticals in specific cases and set standards of medical treatment, taking into account their costs, work on these formularies has not been completed. Meanwhile, there are therapeutic committees in most hospitals that develop hospital formularies containing list of pharmaceuticals used in a particular hospital and information on the restrictions in their use. Moreover, prescribing of reimbursed pharmaceuticals is monitored by the NFZ. It is used for controlling potential abuses rather than as a criterion for selecting healthcare providers for NFZ's contracts [7].

Ukraine

Pricing of Pharmaceuticals

The State Expert Centre (until 27 September 2010 called the State Pharmacological Centre) and the State Administration of Ukraine on Medicinal Products (SAUMP) are the main two regulatory bodies for pharmaceuticals both of which are under Ministry of Health. The State Expert Centre is responsible for the registration and quality control of pharmaceuticals, preclinical, clinical and post clinical research; monitoring adverse drug reactions (although adverse drug reaction reporting by physicians is very low); developing the list of pharmaceuticals that may be bought over the counter and submitting it for approval to the Ministry of Health; authorizing the import and use of unregistered pharmaceuticals; advising on the content of the National Drug Formulary and standardizing medical services, including pharmaceutical services (8).

According to the laws, pharmaceuticals are allowed to be used after the registration process in which preclinical examinations and clinical trial results are required to be presented to ensure the quality and safety. Registration process is carried out by State Expert Centre [8].

Upon with the Law on pharmaceuticals in Ukraine, amended on 5 September 2014, the pharmaceuticals indicated in tuberculosis, HIV/AIDS, cancer and rare diseases are subjected to a simplified marketing authorization process which means fast-track registration of pharmaceuticals that have been approved by competent authorities of the United States of America, Swiss Confederation, Japan, Australia, New Zealand, Canada, the EU or Israel (countries with "high regulatory standards") [8].

There is a negative list consisting of pharmaceuticals that can be sold without a prescription and pharmaceuticals out of this negative list are nominally sold only with prescription. Although MoH prepares a list of prescription only pharmaceuticals, most of them may be bought over the counter. On the other hand, pharmacies strictly control the supply of psychotropic drugs and hormonal preparations, even though many others, such as antibiotics, can usually be bought without a prescription.

In 2003 a national program that outlines the selection of safe and efficient use of pharmaceuticals by using pharmacoeconomic analysis was developed for the period between 2004 and 2010 in order to improve pharmaceuticals provision. By this program a formulary-based drug procurement system was introduced in order to improve tender procedures for state purchases of pharmaceuticals, to identify state priorities for pharmaceutical purchasing, improve the quality of treatment and provide clinicians with access to information on the use of pharmaceuticals registered in Ukraine. This program also included the state registration of wholesale prices, the introduction of appropriate laboratory, clinical, industrial and distribution practices based on such standards as GMP and good laboratory practice (GLP). A list of essential pharmaceuticals was also approved in accordance with the program.

The main direct mechanism of state price regulation of pharmaceuticals is based on establishing maximum retail surcharges. Due to the decentralized regulation approach, retail surcharges, retail and wholesale prices differ substantially between different regions.

Before 2008, there were 149 international nonproprietary names of pharmaceuticals from various clinical and pharmacological groups in the list of pharmaceuticals subject to state price regulation and they constituted 21% of the Essential Drug List. On November 2001 due to the amendments on certain decrees of the Cabinet of Ministers, a maximum limit of retail surcharges at the national level for these pharmaceuticals is determined which is 35% of the manufacturer's wholesale price (customs cost) distributed through the pharmacy network; and 10% for products that are purchased by publicly owned healthcare facilities with funds allocated from the budget.

In 2008, by the initiation of the global financial crisis, pharmaceutical prices have increased substantially (by 40-70%) due to the currency devaluation. In relation with this fact, government adopted a series of cost containment measures such as expanding the list of pharmaceuticals subject to state price regulation to cover almost the entire Essential Medicines List – 903 generic drugs (or 85% of all registered drugs in Ukraine). The mark-up limits were set at no more than 10% of wholesale prices and 25% of retail price; for pharmaceuticals purchased through the budget the mark-up limit was set at 10% of wholesale and 10% of retail price. As a result of this amendment, the range of pharmaceuticals available in pharmacies was reduced, the social tension was increased and pharmaceutical industry showed resistance by stating that they faced bankruptcy.

In 2009, state price controls of pharmaceuticals softened with a decree and in 2010, this decree was transformed into a mechanism that controls the wholesale prices of pharmaceuticals purchased through the state and local budgets.

Since 2012, a pilot project that initiates state price regulation for essential antihypertensive pharmaceuticals, using reference pricing mechanisms and reimbursement has started to be applied. All generic antihypertensive pharmaceuticals that are priced at or below the maximum wholesale price level are divided into three groups: those reimbursed at 90% of the reference price; those reimbursed at up to 90%; and those that are not reimbursed. In this context, prescribed antihypertensive pharmaceuticals are distributed by healthcare facilities and pharmacies listed by the regional health authorities and after patients pay the difference between the actual retail price and the reference price as approved by the MoH. However, these measures did not reach its goal and retail prices have increased above the rate of inflation. As reimbursement covered the locally produced generics, the price of antihypertensive pharmaceuticals on the market was reduced by 9.3% and the consumption increased by 24%. Although prices in the pharmaceuticals market have stabilized to some extent, the government system for price controls remains an inefficient aspect of the pharmaceuticals supply chain.

There are four price control lists:
- National List;
- List of drugs that can be purchased through local or state budgets;
- Mandatory minimum range of socially important pharmaceuticals and medical products;
- List of pharmaceuticals covered by the pilot project on hypertension.

Presence of number of lists leads significant amount of duplication that results in higher prices. In addition, although the declared price system provides formal declaration procedures for the manufacturers/importers, accurate and objective information on the prices declared by the state are not checked. As the control of compliance with the mandated mark-up levels are not performed effectively by the state, 76% of the cost of a pharmaceutical goes directly to the manufacturer/importer [8].

Reimbursement of Pharmaceuticals

Outpatients and sometimes even inpatients are obliged to pay for drugs out of pocket except some certain groups. Certain population groups including vulnerable population groups and patients with socially significant and very serious diseases, such as tuberculosis, cancer, etc., are entitled to some benefits in receiving medical services and pharmaceuticals. They are may receive pharmaceuticals services either free of charge or with significant discounts. These benefits mostly include outpatient drugs. Drugs prescribed for outpatients that are on the government-approved list must be provided free or with discounts. Benefits-related pharmaceutical costs are meant to be covered by state budget allocations to healthcare. However in practice, even vulnerable population groups have to pay for pharmaceuticals out of pocket most of the time.

As stated above, since 2012 a pilot project has been in place regarding pricing and reimbursement of antihypertensive pharmaceuticals. These kinds of schemes are expected to be extended for other pharmaceutical groups especially for insulin [8,11].

5.3 Mapping and Structure of Decision Makers

Russia

The main regulatory bodies for pharmaceuticals are MoH, the Ministry of Industry and Trade (MIT) and Federal service for Surveillance in Healthcare [6].

The main responsibilities of MoH include determining the state policy and regulations related with health and circulation of pharmaceuticals for human use. MoH implements majority of important executive regulations on the circulation of pharmaceuticals required by laws and presents drafts of federal laws on health.

MoH's activities cover:
- Adaptation of general pharmacopoeial monographs and publishing the state pharmacopoeia;
- Registration of pharmaceuticals for human use;
- Emitting the permits for the conduct of clinical trials;
- Emitting the permits for the importation of a specific batch of unregistered pharmaceuticals for clinical trials, for expert examination for the purposes of state registration, and for rendering medical aid to a patient if he or she has extremely serious indications;
- Registration of maximum manufacturers' prices of pharmaceuticals included in the list of essential and most important pharmaceuticals, also known as the Essential Drug List (EDL)

MIT's activities cover:
- Playing an important role in the procedure for declaration of conformity and certification of medicinal preparations;
- Granting the licenses for the manufacture of pharmaceuticals;
- Registration of licenses granted.

Federal Service's activities cover:
- Controlling the circulation of pharmaceuticals by means of inspections on compliance with the rules on laboratory and clinical practices while performing pre-clinical trials of pharmaceuticals and clinical trials of medicinal preparations, rules on man-

ufacturing and quality control, rules on wholesale trade of pharmaceuticals, dispensing rules and rules on production of medicinal preparations and rules on the storage and destruction of pharmaceuticals;

- Controlling the quality of pharmaceuticals;
- Controlling the prices of EDL medicinal preparations;
- Monitoring the assortment and prices of EDL medicinal preparations;
- Monitoring the safety of medicinal preparations;
- Granting licenses for pharmaceutical activities;
- Registration of licenses granted;
- Controlling the quality and safety of medical activity through inspections of the compliance of medical professionals, heads of medical organizations, pharmaceutical professionals and heads of pharmacies with applicable professional guidelines.

Poland

The Ministry of Health

Since 1989, the role of the MoH has progressively evolved from the funder and organizer of healthcare provision to policymaker and regulator [7].

MoH's main responsibilities include:
- Governance and organization of healthcare sector;
- National health policy, implementation and coordination of health policy programs;
- Management of major capital investments;
- Medical research and education (the Ministry has administrative responsibility only for the institutions that it finances directly from the part of the state budget allocated to health, including the Medical Centre of Postgraduate Education (*Centrum Medyczne Kształcenia Podyplomowego* – CMKP, the Institute of Mother and Child and Institute of Cardiology);
- Semi-autonomous medical academies, university hospitals and research institutes;
- Supervision of the training of healthcare personnel;
- Funding very expensive medical equipment (the responsibility in this area is shared with territorial self-governments);
- Determination and monitoring of healthcare standards;
- Funding of certain emergency medical services;
- Confirmation of regional medical emergency care plans prepared by the *voivodes*;
- Development of guidelines for health promotion and disease prevention programs;
- Elaboration of solutions to health problems caused by environmental and social factors, and jointly with the *voivodeships*, evaluation of access to healthcare;
- Supervision of the Chief Pharmaceutical Inspectorate (*Główny Inspektorat Farmaceutyczny*), the Office for Registration of Medicinal Products, Medical Devices and Biocides (*Urząd Rejestracji Produktów Leczniczych, Wyrobów Medycznych i Produktów Biobójczych* – URPL,WMiPB) and the Chief.

The National Health Fund (Narodowy Fundusz Zdrowia (NFZ))

Funding of healthcare services is the main responsibility of NFZ.

NFZ's main responsibilities include:

- Funding and implementation of healthcare programs;
- Negotiation of contracts for service provision with healthcare providers;
- Monitoring the fulfillment of contractual terms that influence the quality and accessibility of healthcare services to a certain extent;
- Covering the costs of healthcare services provided in other EU Member States to Polish citizens;
- Promotion of health;
- Monitoring of medical prescribing;
- Maintaining the Central Registry of Insured Persons.

Engagement in profit-making activities and operating own or co-own healthcare institutions are forbidden for NFZ. NFZ has a council supervising the its activities and a president ensuring the management and representation. Council and the Parliamentary Commission for Health and the Parliamentary Commission for Public Finance of the Sejm determine the annual financial plan for NFZ. This plan is required to be approved the Ministry of Health in consultation with the Ministry of Finance [7].

Professional chambers

Physicians, dentists, pharmacists, nurses and midwives and laboratory diagnosticians are associated in professional chambers. They provide expert opinion or arbitrate on issues of professional responsibility and supervise healthcare services. Professional chambers contribute establishment of education standards, maintain registers of licensed and active professionals and monitor their participation in continuous education. Membership in the chambers is compulsory for all practicing professionals [7].

The National Institute of Public Health

The National Institute of Public Health–National Institute of Hygiene (*Narodowy Instytut Zdrowia Publicznego–Państwowy Zakład Higieny* – NIZP-PZH) is responsible for protection of the human population through numerous actions taken in the range of public health, therein science and research works and courses. The activity refers to the monitoring of: biological, chemical and physical risk factors in nutrition, water and air in rooms, as well as contagious diseases and infections. NIPZ-NIH leads expertise activity for the government, non-governmental organizations as well as for the society, within the range of risk assessment and indicating ways for avoiding threats. Institute also leads researches of the vaccines quality [7].

The National Agency for Health Technology Assessment and Tarification (AHTAPol)

Established in 2005, AHTAPol is the first public entity in the Polish healthcare system whose main activity was the assessment of technologies financed by public. AHTAPol serves as an advisory body to the MoH to inform decisions on public funding of health technologies, particularly those that are included in the basic benefits package besides NFZ and Quality Monitoring Center.

The most important tasks of AHTAPol include healthcare services, pharmaceuticals and medical devices and healthcare programs. Regarding to healthcare services, AHTAPol make recommendations related with the determination of their inclusion/exclusion in the basket of guaranteed services and the level or methodology of financing or the conditions of services. Regarding to pharmaceuticals and medical devices, AHTAPol make recommendations related with the determination of their inclusion in the basket of guaranteed services. Regarding to healthcare governmental health programs, AHTAPol makes assessments.

The Agency's main role is to assess the pharmaceuticals and describe the services. Pharmaceutical companies must submit an application dossier to ATHAPol in parallel to the one submitted to MoH containing a full HTA report analyzing clinical effectiveness, cost-effectiveness and budget impact. The report is then critically assessed by an analytical team at AHTAPol, according to a set of HTA guidelines elaborated by a team of experts under the auspices of the AHTAPol [12]. Assessment procedure includes the evaluation of submitted evidence, search of new available evidence, revision of the economic analysis and validation of costs economic modeling and budget impact analysis. Agency also refers to key clinical experts and NFZ. The applicant has the right to comment to the assessment of the Agency. Taking both into consideration the assessment and the comments, Transparence Council of the AHTAPol structures the final opinion, which constitutes the basis of the recommendation presented to MoH. AHTAPol's recommendations are not legally binding and the MoH always makes the final decision.

Besides AHTAPol, in 2007 the Transparence Council is established as an another HTA agency [7].

Ukraine

The central government, the Ministry of Finance, the Ministry of Health (MoH) and local governments are the main regulatory bodies in Ukrainian Health system. "Parliament sets the goals, major objectives, priorities, budget guidelines and regulatory framework for the health sector, and approves the targeted national health programs. The President is responsible for ensuring that health policy is implemented in accordance with legislation and the Constitution through the system of executive bodies. The Cabinet of Ministers coordinates the development and implementation of national programs and creates legal, economic and managerial mechanisms to support the health system"[8].

The Ministry of Finance (MoF) is responsible for the preparation of the draft state budget that indicates the public resources to be allocated to the health sector in any given year. MoF also determines the requirements for state institutions (including healthcare facilities) in formulating and implementing budgets [8].

MoH manages the healthcare system over 24 regional administrations and two city-states administrations located in Sevastopol and Kyiv. MoH develops and implements national health policies including the policies on specific diseases like HIV and funds certain publicly owned healthcare institutions specialized in certain diseases, research institutes, higher medical educational establishments, research institutes, and publicly owned medico-prophylactic facilities at the national level. MoH is also responsible for controlling the significant proportions of the centralized state purchase of pharmaceuticals, medical devices and equipment for the relevant state programs [8]. "The Ministry of Labor and Social Policy is responsible, among other things, for overseeing the provision of long-term residential care for elderly people and people with disabilities" [8]. The National Academy of Medical Sciences is responsible for provision of highly specialized medical services.

There are many non-governmental organizations (NGOs) consisting of professional medical associations and patient groups, which are actively working and becoming more influential [8].

5.4 Challenges and Catalyzers for Market Access

Russia

Challenges

Russia imposes international reference pricing based on the lowest price in the basket of reference countries. According to the Pharmaceutical Research and Manufacturers of America (PhRMA) report, this system is suboptimal as it incorrectly assumes that the economic conditions, patient populations and needs and healthcare systems in the reference countries are relevant to Russia. PhRMA and its member companies believe that Russia should adopt a pricing and reimbursement system that appropriately values and rewards innovation [13].

With regard to the "Development trends and practical aspects of the Russian pharmaceutical industry - 2015" report of Deloitte based on the opinions of the respondents representing foreign companies engaged in the production of original pharmaceuticals in Russia and abroad and those of industry experts and analysts; the most serious problems faced by pharmaceutical and healthcare companies in Russia are defined as [14]:

- 26% of the respondents stated economic situation and lack of solvency among individuals;
- 24% of the respondents stated shortcomings in the sector's legal regulation including pricing, antimonopoly, administrative, etc.;
- 15% of the respondents stated lack of state funding for healthcare programs and support for Russian manufacturers;
- 14% of the respondents stated the current geopolitical situation, related economic risks and negative consequences for Russian manufacturers;
- 6% of the respondents stated corruption;
- 5% of the respondents stated the increased competition in the market.

Catalyzers

According to the ¨Unlocking Pharma Growth¨ report of McKinsey published in 2012 Russian pharmaceutical market offers important opportunities in the next decade as the value of the market grows from $15 billion to $41 billion by 2020. The growth is likely to be based on all channels. In this regard, the fastest growth is expected to come from the state funded channels with their share of the market to be increased from 36% to 42% by 2020 [15]. In the next three to five years a new state funded national drug insurance program for the general population is expected to be introduced and accordingly the government spending on health is expected to increase. Out of pocket spending may also rise due to the rapid expansion of middle class: by 2015 the proportion of households with annual incomes above $10,000 is expected to rise from 35 percent to roughly 50 percent [15].

Corresponding with the Healthcare 2020 development strategy, live expectancy is aimed to increase to 75 years. This would increase the government spending on healthcare [15].

Poland

Challengers

According to the Investing in Poland, 2014 report, the reimbursement Act, came to force in January 2012, has affected the pharmaceutical market including patients, doctors, producers, wholesalers and pharmacies [16]. Law on the Reimbursement of Drugs, Food for Special Medical Purposes (FSMPs) and Medical Devices from 2011 was the first piece of legislation in the history of that collected together and systematized the process of reimbursement in Poland. The law's main effect was to lower the price limits for reimbursed drugs so that savings could be used for the introduction of innovative drugs into the system.

The new law has created many benefits and also many victims, causing bankruptcies and lay-offs. "Many pharmacies, especially those with large shares of reimbursed drugs in their turnover, have felt the pain" said Tomasz Dzitko, chairman of the pharmaceutical committee at the Business Centre Club, Poland's largest employer organization. "Prices of a number of innovative, reimbursed drugs were cut to levels that made sales hardly profitable" said Ms Stefańczyk. Some drugs were completely removed from the outpatient sector's reimbursement lists [16].

That's one of the reasons why Poland's entire pharmaceutical market has shrunk. "The number of employees fell by more than 9 percent" said Dr Dariusz Nowicki, director of the Polish Chamber of Pharmaceutical Industries and Medical Devices Polfarmed. "The net profits for the whole sector dropped by almost half in 2012. Investment outlays decreased by more than 30 percent same year, compared with two years back. Total wholesale margins were drop further in 2014 from 9.8 percent in 2012 to just 5 percent according to Mr Dzitko" [16].

Catalyzers

According to the McKinsey's report published in January 2015, Poland could become a pharmaceutical hub for Europe or even globally, by developing capabilities as a manufacturing center for complex generics and biosimilars. It also has the potential to strengthen its role as a manufacturing contractor for European generic products and become a packaging and logistics center for the European pharmaceutical industry [17].

"The pharmaceuticals market in Poland has grown continuously for the last decade and now accounts for around 1 percent of GDP. The market is the largest in Central Europe and the sixth largest in the European Union. Pharmaceutical exports, especially to Western Europe, have been strong and on the rise, as local producers have increased their focus on more advanced-medicine markets. According to McKinsey estimates, the value-added breakdown in pharmaceuticals ranges from 70 to 90 percent in manufacturing, with up to 15 percent in distribution and 3 to 5 percent in logistics. Poland has established a solid reputation and the fundamentals in the manufacture and marketing of pharmaceutical products. Strengths include generic prescription drugs (branded and non-branded as contract manufacturing) and branded over-the-counter (OTC) products. Production reached EUR 2.8 billion in 2013, reflecting 6 percent annual growth. Several modern manufacturing plants are operating in the sector, with skilled labor that is competitive with specialists from other countries. The plants are situated in attractive locations, furthermore, to serve extensive Western, Central, and Eastern European geographies" [17].

According to the Poland: Eastern Europe's Leading Light report published in June 2015, Poland's central location, stable economy, highly qualified staff and strong government incentives make Poland a very attractive market for pharmaceuticals [18]. Highlights of this report are listed below.

- Poland's stability and bright outlook attracts most global pharmaceutical companies. Many pharmaceutical companies have their central and eastern European headquarters in Poland.
- Poland's location makes it ideal for exporting products to Europe and Asia, its economy is stable and there are many incentives to bolster the market.
- Authorities have created 14 Special Economic Zones to encourage and facilitate development of new companies and to offer tax incentives along with additional funds.
- Biotech sector which is one of the fastest growing factors in Poland, has easy access to government grants, EU funds and tax incentives.
- Poland has the ability to compete with low cost countries through stability, economic development and by investing in potential candidates and professionals.
- Poland has a well-developed manufacturing infrastructure, logistics and know-how and very strong network of scientific institutes.
- While the Polish pharmaceutical market has largely consisted of high-volume generics, a number of Polish companies have started R&D operations focused on novel molecules, innovative therapies, and biosimilar products. According to the Central Office of Statics of Poland, in 2013 there were 191 companies in Poland conducting R&D in biotechnology.

- Poland is the largest clinical trials market in CEE (Central and Eastern Europe)/CIS (Commonwealth of independent States) and accounts for roughly 20% of the clinical trials in Eastern Europe. More than 400 studies are registered in Poland every year.
- Poland's regulatory processes are predictable and transparent. Poland doesn't have major corruption issues, investigators are experienced, logistics are easy and improving and the costs remain lower than in western European countries or North America.

Ukraine

Challenges

Intellectual Property Protections

- **Compulsory Licensing Resolution.** On December 4, 2013, the Cabinet of Ministers adopted a resolution on approval of the procedure for granting authorization to use an object of intellectual property regarding a medicinal product by the cabinet of ministers of Ukraine. According to the PhRMA's Special 301 Submission 2013, although representatives of the research-based pharmaceutical industry were included and propose several amendments in the process, the contours of the proposed compulsory licensing mechanism remain uncertain. Related with this fact, PhRMA and its member companies are highly concerned that Ukraine could issue compulsory licenses in order to support the commercial interests of specific local companies to the detriment of U.S. manufacturers of innovative pharmaceuticals [19].

Market access barriers

- **Price regulation measures.** In May 2013, as the Cabinet of Ministers of Ukraine amended a resolution on a pilot project on state price regulation for anti-hypertensive medicines. Most imported anti-hypertensive medicines are excluded from Ukraine's reimbursement lists. On August 2013, another Pilot Project on state price regulation for insulin products was launched by the Cabinet of Ministers. The reference pricing methodology proposed by the Ministry of Health (MoH) may challenge the insulin sales of the research-based pharmaceutical industry [19].
- **Import Licensing.** In July 2012, the amendment of the law regarding to licensing imports of pharmaceuticals and defining the term active pharmaceutical ingredient (API) was adopted. In accordance with this amendment, in May 2013, Import Licensing Conditions is developed by MoH and become valid through December 2013. Despite the conditions were supposed to administer similar standards with EU standards, the differences between EU and Ukraine wasn't successfully taken into account in terms of importation systems, laboratory capacity and distribution models. As a result of the negotiations of pharmaceutical industry with the State Administration on pharmaceuticals between July and November 2013, amendments on the import licensing conditions that delays some of the less-defined aspects of the Conditions until March 2016 was adopted at the end of 2013. In this regard, according to

PhRMA members, there may be some discriminations against foreign manufacturers compared to local manufacturers which will not have to obtain a similar license [19].

Catalyzers

On September 2014, Ukrainian and European parliaments signed the EU–Ukraine Association Agreement (AA) that provides harmonization of many spheres of Ukrainian legislation with EU policy. In this regard, the government has adopted a detailed implementation plan for a new healthcare system in Ukraine to be prepared and approved by the end of 2015. The plan covers all fields of the healthcare sector including financing public hospitals and reimbursement of pharmaceuticals and medical devices with the long-term goal of establishing a developed and sustainable regulatory framework in Ukraine [20].

On September 2014, a category of products subjected to simplified marketing authorization procedures was submitted with an amendment on Law on pharmaceuticals. This category of products covers tuberculosis, HIV/AIDS, cancer and rare diseases' pharmaceuticals and the pharmaceuticals that are authorized by competent authorities of the United States, Swiss Confederation, Japan, Australia, Canada or European Union [20].

Due to the facts that there is an emerging political consensus on the need to introduce reimbursement and an insurance-based healthcare system and aging population and demographic trends, the pharmaceutical expenditures are expected to rise in the long term and the pharmaceutical market is expected to remain attractive. Sub-sector best prospects include: analgesics and antibiotics, anti-cancer pharmaceuticals, vaccines, cough and cold preparations, vaso-therapeutics and hemostatic agents [21].

As being highly flexible and positively evaluated for investment, the Ukrainian pharmaceutical market is among the fastest moving pharmaceutical markets in Europe accordingly. As there is no significant global player operating in the Ukraine currently, entering the Ukrainian pharmaceutical market can be facilitated for potential investors resulting in a less competitive market sector.

Besides the investment and market opportunities, Ukraine is a good location for exporting to the other eastern countries such as Uzbekistan and Kazakhstan, where in such less developed countries, the current demand outstrips the available opportunities [22].

5.5 Good Examples from Successful Market Access Strategies

Russia

- Majority of the pharmaceutical companies operating in the emerging markets canalizes their efforts of sales and marketing to physicians and hospitals. However, recently, in order to address a large and neglected opportunity, companies build retail arm. In this regard, in Russia, distributers have more influence on the retail channel than pharmacies do. As an example, CV Protek, one of the country's largest distributors, made a forward integration with Rigla, a leading pharmacy chain [15].

- In recent years multinational companies (MNCs) have significantly increased their investments in emerging markets and especially the large middle-income markets. In Russia, Glaxo Smith Kline supplies bulk vaccines and provides technology and expertise to Binnopharm, which then undertakes the filling and packaging in order to become a part of the national immunization calendar. The agreement includes the pharmaceuticals of oncology, rotavirus and pneumococcal vaccines. Related with the same aim, Pfizer and NPO Petrovax Pharm have been co-manufacturing pneumococcal vaccine since 2011 and Pfizer provides technology transfer and expertise to increase production quality among local producers, in accordance with GMP standards [23].
- Some companies make collaborations with local technology platforms in high incidence areas to secure future revenues by driving R&D investments on specific diseases. As an example, Roche enter into a partnership with ChemRar on anti-thrombotic agents in Russia. Some other companies help to address local needs while developing technology with the potential to be applied globally. For instance, Genzyme works with ChemRar to develop vaccines for orphan diseases by using genetic modification technologies to deliver personalized pharmaceuticals [15].
- Public private partnerships are becoming more widespread due to the increase in the competition in emerging markets. In Russia, Novartis worked directly with members of the cabinet to understand their needs. It was then able to raise its public profile and market visibility with a $500 million pledge to invest in new R&D centers in Skolkovo, in a direct response to President Medvedev's plan to create a world-class biotech cluster [15].

Poland

According to the PwC's report called Impact of the Innovative Pharma Industry on the Polish Economy; over half of the TOP 30 pharma companies operating on the Polish market have production facilities in Poland. The three largest companies in Poland are innovative pharma players with production facilities (Novartis, Sanofi-Aventis and GSK).

"Undoubtedly, the range of interactions within the domestic economy increases alongside rising investments. Some pharma companies have their production facilities in different regions of Poland. Moreover, some innovative pharma companies have also established their functional hubs in Poland (e.g. IT, Clinical Research and Shared Service Centers). Market feedback indicates the absence of incentives supporting the development of investments at the central government level. However, overall cooperation with local authorities is very highly rated" [24].

In recent years big pharmaceutical companies have put significant effort into setting up dedicated units with a brief to improve interactions with academics, Examples include the Johnson & Johnson innovation centers, Pfizer's Centers for Therapeutic Innovation (CTI) and GSK's DPAc program [25].

- "Johnson & Johnson Innovation represents a new approach to partnering aimed at advancing early-stage innovation. Johnson & Johnson's teams of science and business experts, based in regional innovation centers, collaborate with innovators to accelerate cutting edge science into healthcare solutions" [26].

- "Launched in 2010, Pfizer's Centers for Therapeutic Innovation (CTI) is a model for academic-industry collaboration, designed to bridge the gap between early scientific discovery and its translation into new medicines. A key aspect of CTI is its local Centers in biomedical research hubs that enable Pfizer and academic teams to work side-by-side, blending the research expertise of academics in disease biology, targets, and patient populations with Pfizer's developmental expertise and resources. This model represents a significant departure from the traditional lengthy and linear process of target discovery to eventual drug development. Pfizer funds pre-clinical and clinical development programs and offers equitable intellectual property and ownership rights and access to antibody libraries and other proprietary technologies" [27].
- "GSK has established DPAc to bring together the insight of the academic world with the complementary expertise and capabilities of GSK in joint, target-focused, early drug discovery projects. DPAc looks for partners who really want to be involved in developing a medicine. Suitable projects have a compelling therapeutic hypothesis and are at a stage where partnership with GSK will make a key contribution to success. GSK applies resources to these projects, including development of robust assays, lead identification using conventional screening, rational design, encoded libraries and biological therapeutic optimization, medicinal chemistry and preclinical development. This work is integrated with activities ongoing in the academic groups" [28].

Ukraine

GlaxoSmithKline in cooperation with the Ministry of Health and respected NGO partners, PBN Hill+Knowlton Strategies conducted an educational campaign targeting the general media and women with the aim of educating women about cervical cancer and new preventive methods and creating a public dialogue on the issues in Ukraine. This campaign succeeded in increasing awareness among target audiences about cervical cancer prevention methods through the distribution of printed materials in hospitals, private clinics, women's health consultancies and other institutions and through generating extensive coverage in the general media and women's magazines [29].

Roche has expanded differential pricing program in Ukraine to co-develop methods for evaluating the medical value and benefit of new pharmaceuticals and diagnostics, negotiate commercial arrangements that improve access to Roche products, co-develop flexible pricing models to address affordability across the different regions and jointly develop tailored programs with government to strengthen healthcare infrastructure [30].

5.6 Look up for near future

Russia

In 2009, Russia adopted the strategy for development of the Pharmaceutical industry by 2020, known as "Pharma 2020". The main objective of the Russian state policy regarding the development of national pharmaceutical industry for the period up to 2020 is creating conditions for the transition of the Russian pharmaceutical production towards an innovative development model [31].

The main objectives of the strategy are mentioned as [31]:

1. Increase the supply of nationally-produced essential and rare-disease treatment medication for the Russian population, the healthcare system institutions, the defense sector and other related federal services;
2. Improve the competitiveness of the domestic pharmaceutical industry by synchronizing the Russian standards of medication development and production with international requirements;
3. Stimulate the development and production of innovative medication;
4. Protect the internal market from unfair competition and provide equal access conditions for domestic and foreign producers;
5. Technically re-equip the Russian pharmaceutical industry;
6. Enhancement of the system of quality conformity of medication, including measures to eliminate excessive administrative barriers during registration of domestic drugs;
7. Prepare specialists for the pharmaceutical production design and manufacturing in compliance with international standards.

Expected final results of the strategy implementations are mentioned as [31]:

- Increase of the domestic products share to 50% of the total in the internal market (in value terms) by 2020;
- Change the range of medication manufactured in Russia, including an increase of innovative products up to 60% in value terms;
- Increase the export of pharmaceutical products by 8 times compared to 2008;
- Guarantee of safety and compliance of drugs with the list of strategically-important drugs in the Russian Federation;
- Stimulate the establishment of pharmaceutical productions on Russian territory in the volumes necessary for an output of 50% of finished substances (in value terms), including no less than 85% of drugs listed in VDL.

Another important program of the Russian pharmaceutical market and SREW (Scientific research and experimental works) development is the "Comprehensive developmental program of biotechnologies in Russia up to 2020". The Ministry of Economic Development is the coordinator of this program.

The main objective is the creation of a competitive sector of bio-economy. The need for such a program is caused by Russia's very low share in the world biotechnological market, especially due to low degree of commercialization of scientific research; a high demand in imports; the current international tendency to replace chemical products with biological ones; and opportunities to recycle agro-industrial wastes.

In addition to measures that are planned under "Pharma-2020" Strategy, it is also needed to implement the following measures for the support of biotechnological development as [31]:

- Stimulating the demand for biotechnological production through development of an appropriate regulatory framework, formation of state procurement mechanisms, improvement of legal support for biomedical products and services, circulation and other measures;

- Assisting biotechnological companies through the growing competitiveness via grants, improving export system and the support for the import of new technologies;
- Scientific development in biotechnology which includes the development of research programs in individual segments of biotechnology including medicine as well as improving the competitive selection mechanism and simplification of tender procedures;
- Creation of an information-analysis infrastructure within which it is planned to develop a biotechnological network that would connect the industry's organizations and structures; creation of a knowledge base; creating of a the system for the monitoring of the program implementation process.

The expected results of the program include a new level of biotechnological production in Russia, which will reach 1% of GDP by 2020.

The implementation of the Strategy for the development of the national pharmaceutical sector should help return investments to the industry by 2017, due to discounts on generic and innovative products manufactured in Russia, provided by budgetary funds as well as by additional tax revenues from the income of local pharmaceutical manufacturers.

Poland

According to the Poland 2025 report of McKinsey & Company published in 2015, in the nearest future, Poland is expected to have a "R&D boom" and pharmaceutical sector is among the most popular areas of R&D activities [17].

Apart from R&D activities, considering the whole healthcare system, as a result of the elections of Poland parliamentary held on 25 October 2015, by the replacement of the liberal-conservative Civic Platform (Platform Obywatelska; PO) by conservative Law and Justice (Prawo i Sprawiedliwość; PiS) significant changes are expected to be implemented in the Poland's healthcare system and pharmaceutical policy.

With reference to IHS, it is unclear whether PiS government will carry on with PO's pharmaceutical policy. It is stated that "For public healthcare in general, PiS has set an agenda which includes proposals for some very fundamental changes to the entire public healthcare infrastructure in Poland. The most high-profile pledge given by PiS regarding healthcare is that it will abolish the National Health Fund (NFZ). As well as this, PiS plans to get rid of mandatory health insurance contributions, transferring the responsibility for funding public healthcare to the state budget. However, there are serious questions about what PiS plans to replace the NFZ with. The process of contracting healthcare services is set to be taken over by voivodeship (regional) governments, and the administrative complications and costs of this process could be significant. And, in the end, it will still be an 'official' in a public body making the decisions. The contracting activities include contracting for hospital services, which includes the funds required for hospital drugs, including high-cost drugs. However, PiS intends to divide the public healthcare budget so that most services will be paid for at the regional level, but highly specialized services and high-cost, modern medical technologies will be paid for centrally by the Ministry of Health (MoH) – including presumably high-cost innovative medicines. What the implications of such a change would be are hard to predict – if this means a closed, separate budget for high-cost and highly-specialized medicine, there could be problems with access to medicines once the budget is exhausted" [32].

"PiS politicians have stated their intention also to raise the proportion of GDP spent on public healthcare in Poland from the current level of around 4.7% to 6%. Konstanty Radziwiłł, a medical doctor and former head of Poland's Supreme Medical Council who has been announced as the new government's health minister, has stated that this goal of 6% of GDP should be reached within 2-3 years. If these were to actually happen, and the extra funds were allocated fairly and evenly, this would, of course, be a very positive thing. However, considering the fact that PiS has made a series of promises –including a policy of PLN500 per month for families who have second, third or more children (as well as for the poorest families with only one child) and a reduction of the retirement age back to 65 for women and 60 for men – that are estimated by experts to cost an additional PLN55 billion per year to implement, it is worth asking where the extra money to make this increase in healthcare spending will come from" [32].

"Another plan, which has featured prominently in PiS' campaign, is the introduction of free medicines for poorer pensioners aged over 75 years" [32].

Ukraine

In 2015, Strategic Advisory Group on healthcare reform of Ukraine has published a report called National Health Reform Strategy for Ukraine 2015-2020 that sets the context, vision, principles, priorities, objectives and key measures in the Ukrainian health system in the coming period [33].

Regarding pharmaceutical sector, following goals are aimed to be achieved:
- Ensuring pharmaceuticals and health products to be safe, affordable and effective;
- Being compliant with the standards, rules and norms in accordance with the principles of good practices in pharmaceuticals as per EU regulations;
- Introducing the mechanism of mutual recognition of registration dossier assessment for the pharmaceuticals that have registered by National Drug Regulatory Authorities (NDRAs) in United States, Switzerland, Japan, Australia, Canada and the European Union;
- Applying the mutual recognition and parallel import agreement widely in EU countries in pharmaceutical market;
- Facilitating new companies entrance to the Ukrainian Market by reducing bureaucratic and legal barriers;
- Simplifying the GMP certification procedures as favored by Ukraine's membership in PIC/S (the Pharmaceutical Inspection Convention and Pharmaceutical Inspection Co-operation Scheme).

These arrangements would allow implementing free competition on an open market with sufficient safety reassurance. Considering the economic problems and the importance of domestic manufacturing, introducing market liberalization would make price controls of pharmaceuticals an excessive policy instrument.

As mentioned in the report, during the transition period, state prices regulation mechanism could be maintained by using National Essential Pharmaceuticals List which should improve over the implementation of the reform by:

- Introduction of price registration procedures in accordance with EU requirements;
- External price referencing – for original pharmaceuticals; Competitive Price referencing – for generics;
- Launching price reimbursement based on internal prices referencing;
- Monitoring the availability and accessibility of medicines in Ukraine.

National Pharmaceutical Manufacturers will be encouraged to produce pharmaceuticals that are required by the public policy and included into the updated National Essential Pharmaceuticals List. Eventually, electronic tenders and transparent bidding opportunities will apply to international (non-residents of Ukraine) companies, on the same principles that work within the internal pharmaceutical market.

As cited in the report to reduce the cost of pharmaceuticals the state will maintain indirect mechanisms of influence:

- At the physician level (by introducing and improving healthcare protocols and formularies, monitoring drugs consumption, prescribed by doctors, budgeting for reimbursement);
- At the pharmacists level (by supporting generic and therapeutic substitution, falling cost by parallel imports, strengthening pharmacovigilance, etc.);
- At the patients level (by introducing positive and negative reimbursement lists and guaranteed basic package; co-payment promoting, health insurance, including additional medical insurance). For ambulatory sector implementation of the co-payment principles utilizing reimbursement mechanism will become standard procedure in accordance with the requirements of the European Union [33].

5.7 **References**

1. Popovich L, Potapchik E, Shishkin S, et al. Russian Federation: Health system review. *Health Systems in Transition* 2011; 13: 1-190
2. Snapshot report on Russia's healthcare infrastructure industry. Hospital build and infrastructure Russia. Moscow 2013 exhibition and congress
3. Agence wallonne à l'Exportation et aux Investissements Etrangers. Healthcare in Russia. AWEX, 2012. Available at https://www.awex.be/fr-BE/Infos marchés et secteurs/Infossecteurs/Documents/PECO/First DRAFT - копия - копия.rtf (last accessed September 2016)
4. Tarasenko E. Right to health in Russian Federation: identification of its current stage of constitutional and legal recognition. *Revista de Direito Sanitário* 2014; 14: 10-41

5. Räpple T (Ed.). European Pricing and Reimbursement Handbook. 1st edition, Baker & McKenzie, 2011

6. EU Pricing & Reimbursement Pricing & reimbursement schemes in major European countries. Hogan Lovells, 2014

7. Sagan A, Panteli D, Borkowski W, et al. Poland: Health system review. *Health Systems in Transition* 2011; 13: 1-193

8. Lekhan VN, Rudiy VM, Shevchenko MV, et al. Ukraine: Health system review. *Health Systems in Transition* 2015; 17: 1-153

9. Chambers and Partners. Global Practice Guides Life Sciences 2015. Chamber Legal Practice Guides. Available at http://www.chambersandpartners.com/guide/practice-guides/256 (last accessed September 2016)

10. IMS Pharma Pricing & Reimbursement. 2015; 20. Available at https://www.hse.ru/pubs/share/direct/document/145079856 (last accessed September 2016)

11. KPMG Pharma bulletin, Issue #1, 2015 (January). Available at https://home.kpmg.com/ru/en/home/insights/2015/12/kpmg-pharma-bulletin-issue-1.html (last accessed September 2016)

12. Nowakowska E (ed.). Farmakoekonomika [Pharmacoeconomics]. Poznań, Uniwersytetu Medycznego w Poznaniu [Medical University in Poznań], 2010

13. Pharmaceutical Research and Manufacturers of America (PhRMA). Special 301 Submission 2013. Available at http://www.phrma.org/sites/default/files/pdf/PhRMA%20Special%20301%20Submission%202013.pdf (last accessed September 2016)

14. Development trends and practical aspects of the Russian pharmaceutical industry. Deloitte, 2015. Available at http://www2.deloitte.com/content/dam/Deloitte/ru/Documents/life-sciences-health-care/russian-pharmaceutical-industry-2015.pdf (last accessed September 2016)

15. Unlocking pharma growth. Navigating the intricacies of emerging markets. McKinsey & Company, Pharmaceutical and Medical Products Practice 2012. Available at http://www.mckinsey.com/~/media/mckinsey/dotcom/client_service/pharma%20and%20medical%20products/pmp%20new/pdfs/emerging_markets_compendium_2012.ashx (last accessed September 2016)

16. Investing in Poland 2014. Warsaw: Valkea Media, 2014. Available at http://www.pwc.pl/pl/publikacje/assets/investing-in-poland-2014.pdf (last accessed September 2016)

17. Bogdan W, Boniecki D, Labaye E. Poland 2025: Europe's new growth engine. McKinsey & Company, 2015. Available at http://www.mckinsey.com/global-themes/europe/how-poland-can-become-a-european-growth-engine (last accessed September 2016)

18. Ribbink K. Poland: Eastern Europe's Leading Light. PharmaVOICE, 2015. Available at http://www.kcrcro.com/uploads/attachments/news_pdf/PV0615-KCR-Polandv3.pdf (last accessed September 2016)

19. Pharmaceutical Research And Manufacturers of America (PhRMA). Special 301 Submission 2014. Available at http://www.phrma.org/sites/default/files/pdf/2014-special-301-submission.pdf (last accessed September 2016)

20. Sinichkina L, Cherniavskyi L. Market Access in Ukraine. PharmExec.com, 2014. Available at www.pharmexec.com/market-access-ukraine (last accessed September 2016)

21. Export.gov. Ukraine Country Commercial. Helping U.S. Companies Export Guide. 2016. Available at https://www.export.gov/apex/article2?series=a0pt0000000PAv3AAG&type=Country_Commercial__kav (last accessed September 2016)

22. Ukrinvest. Pharmaceutical industry in the Ukraine. Available at http://www.ukrinvest.eu/en/investment-opportunities/pharmaceutical-industry (last accessed September 2016)

23. Buente M, Danner S, Weissbäcker S, et al. Pharma emerging markets 2.0: How emerging markets are driving the transformation of the pharmaceutical industry. Booz & Company, 2013. Available at http://www.strategyand.pwc.com/media/file/Strategyand_Pharma-Emerging-Markets-2.0.pdf (last accessed September 2016)

24. Impact of the Innovative Pharma Industry on the Polish Economy. PwC, 2011. Available at https://www.pwc.pl/pl/publikacje/pwc_impact_of_the_innovative_pharma_industry_on_the_polish_economy.pdf (last accessed September 2016)

25. Zubascu F. Poland making moves to lift barriers to investing in drug discovery. Science|Business, 2015. Available at http://sciencebusiness.net/news/77050/Poland-making-moves-to-lift-barriers-to-investing-in-drug-discovery (last accessed September 2016)

26. Johnson & Johnson Innovation Centers. Available at http://www.jnj.com/partners/innovation-centers

27. Pfizer. Centers for Therapeutic Innovation. Translating Leading Science into Clinical Candidates Through Networked Collaboration. Available at http://www.pfizer.com/research/rd_partnering/centers_for_therapeutic_innovation

28. Center for Research in Molecular Medicine and Chronic Diseases (CiMUS). DPAc Programme Presentation by GSK. Available at http://www.usc.es/cimus/es/events/dpac-programme-presentation-gsk

29. PBN Hill+Knowlton Strategies. GlaxoSmithKline: Cervical Cancer Education in Ukraine. Available at http://pbn-hkstrategies.com/en/Results/GlaxoSmithKline--Cervical-Cancer-Education-in-Ukraine#.Vpircfl97IU (last accessed September 2016)

30. Roche. Stakeholder engagement in 2015. Available at www.roche.com/corp_res_stake_engage.pdf (last accessed September 2016)

31. Russian Pharmaceutical Market. Current review and future outlook until 2020. Opportunities for Swiss companies. OSEC, 2012. Available at http://www.s-ge.com/sites/default/files/private_files/BBK_Russian_Pharmaceutical_Market_Study.pdf (last accessed September 2016)

32. Melck B. Poland's new government – what prospects for healthcare? IHS Markit. Life Sciences Blog 2015. Available at http://blog.ihs.com/poland%E2%80%99s-

new-government-%E2%80%93-what-prospects-for-healthcare (last accessed September 2016)

33. Health Strategic Advisory Group. National Health Reform Strategy for Ukraine 2015-2020. Strategic Advisory Group on healthcare reform of Ukraine, 2015. Available at http://healthsag.org.ua/wp-content/uploads/2015/03/Strategiya_Engl_for_inet.pdf (last accessed September 2016)

Market Access in the United Arab Emirates and Selected Middle Eastern Countries

Ola Ghaleb Al Ahdab

The Middle East

The most widely used geographical definition of the Middle East (ME) states that the Middle East is composed of 18 countries, including Arabic countries and non Arab countries [1].

The Middle Eastern countries are with diverse economies and healthcare systems [2]. The income level and total population in selected Middle East countries are listed in Table 1.

The Gulf Cooperation Council

The Gulf Cooperation Council (GCC), considered part of the ME region, is a regional intergovernmental, political and economic union composed of the following countries: the United Arab Emirates (UAE), Kingdom of Bahrain, Kingdom of Saudi Arabia (KSA), Sultanate of Oman, State of Qatar, State of Kuwait, and the Republic of Yemen (joined in 2003) [3].

The Health Ministers Council of the Arab Countries in the Gulf was established in 1976 as one of the specialized councils in the health field and is based in Riyadh, KSA. In 1991, the name was changed from "Secretariat General Health" (SGH) for the Arab Gulf Cooperation Countries to "The Executive Board of the Health Ministers for Arab GCC" [4].

Country	Region	Income level	GDP (billion US$)	Total population (million)	GDP per capita (US$)
UAE	ME/GCC	High	401.6	9.446	42,515
KSA	ME/GCC	High	746.2	29.37	25,406
Jordan	ME	Upper middle	35.83	6.607	5,423
Egypt	ME	Lower middle	286.5	83.39	3,435
Lebanon	ME	Upper middle	45.73	4.510	1,013

Table 1. World Bank Country Data 2014
GCC = Gulf Cooperation Council; GDP = Gross Domestic Product; KSA = Kingdom of Saudi Arabia; ME = Middle East; UAE = United Arab Emirates

6.2 Introduction

This chapter will discuss healthcare and market access of medicines in selected Middle Eastern countries, focusing on the UAE and highlighting key developments and activities managed and implemented by the GCC Executive Office in the GCC, Saudi Arabia, Jordan, Lebanon, and Egypt.

A general outlook of the healthcare system and health policies in these countries will be introduced. In addition, discussion of the pathways of market access of new medicines including regulation, pricing and reimbursement processes (where applicable), its mapping structure and decision making will be presented. Market access to new medicines can face challenges and have opportunities for catalyzers, examples for successful market access strategies, and where there is possible future adaptation of these strategies will be highlighted.

6.3 General Outlook of Healthcare System and Health Policies in the UAE and Other ME Countries

A general outlook on the healthcare system and structure in selected ME countries will be presented in this section highlighting the key healthcare regulatory bodies and organizations that regulate healthcare delivery in these countries.

The United Arab Emirates (UAE)

The UAE is located in the Gulf Cooperation Council and consists of seven states, termed emirates: Abu Dhabi (the capital), Dubai, Sharjah, Ajman, Umm Al-Quwain, Ras al-Khaimah and Fujairah.

Health problems suffered by the population in the UAE are similar to those of developed countries, a large portion of which are related to sedentary lifestyle, such as metabolic diseases, obesity, diabetes mellitus (DM), asthma, and cancer [5].

The UAE population was estimated at about 9.3 million in 2014 [6], while more than 102 nationalities live in the UAE, UAE nationals represent 19% of the population. The age structure in the UAE shows that the elderly (> 65 years) accounts for about 1% of the population, the 0-14 years category accounts for 20%, while 79% of the population are aged between 15-64 years. Total life expectancy at birth for male/female for the year 2013 is 76/78. The top four leading causes of death reported in the country in 2012 were: ischemic heart disease (17%), road injury (9%), stroke (7%), and congenital anomalies (4%) [5].

The UAE health expenditure share is 20% of the total GCC healthcare expenditure while UAE population share in the GCC is about 12%. Government spending share constitutes 69%, while private sector share is about 31% including out of pocket shares, insurance providers, and nonprofit organizations [7].

	Economy	Score	Previous	Trend
1	Switzerland	5.70	1	
2	Singapore	5.65	2	
3	United States	5.54	5	
4	Finland	5.50	3	
5	Germany	5.49	4	
6	Japan	5.47	9	
7	Hong Kong SAR	5.46	7	
8	Netherlands	5.45	8	
9	United Kingdom	5.41	10	
10	Sweden	5.41	6	
11	Norway	5.35	11	
12	**United Arab Emirates**	**5.33**	**19**	
13	Denmark	5.29	15	

Table 2. Global Competitiveness Report 2014-2015 [14]

In the UAE, the total health expenditure share of Gross Domestic Product (GDP) is 3.3%, and health expenditure *per capita* was reported by UAE national Bureau at US$ 1,639.9 in 2011 [8]. In fact, the WHO country profile shows that the UAE is among the top 20 countries in the world for healthcare spending *per capita* [9]. Drug market expenditure was estimated at US$ bn 1.91 in 2013 [10]. In addition, the UAE tops all other Arab countries in annual *per capita* consumption of medicines [11].

As mentioned earlier, the population structure in the UAE indicates that only 19% are UAE nationals or citizens, the rest are expatriates [12]. This population make up has important consequences for health status and healthcare consumption. The expatriates are often young and stay in the country for a defined period of time.

The healthcare system (HCS) in the UAE is a result of decades of investment in the health sector as depicted in the vision and strategies planned in line with the trends, medical need, and disease burden in the country. Healthcare development and spending are key pursuit in the UAE's ongoing diversification plan. The UAE 2021 vision states that "the UAE will invest continually to build world-class healthcare infrastructure, expertise and services in order to fulfill the citizens' growing needs and expectations" [13]. This is featured in multiple large investments in medical sector technologies and partnerships with international service providers to manage its facilities and aid achieve higher standards in healthcare delivery and infrastructure [9]. As a result, the UAE jumped 7 positions and ranked the 12th globally [14] in the recent Global Competitiveness Report 2014-2015. This report evaluates the ability of 148 countries to provide high levels of prosperity and welfare to its citizens (Table 2).

There are 121 hospitals currently operating throughout the seven Emirates. The World Health Organization 2014 reports state that there are 19.3 physicians and 40.9 nurses and midwives per 10,000 inhabitants and 1.1 beds per 1000 inhabitants in the UAE [12].

The key contributors to the healthcare system are the regulators, providers, payers, and suppliers. The main regulators are the UAE government via federal laws, international obligations, Ministry of Health (MoH) decrees, circulars and standards [15], and local health authorities' standards, i.e. Health Authority Abu Dhabi (HAAD) [16], Dubai Health Authority (DHA) [17], and Sharjah Health Care City [18], which has been recently established.

Health service providers are: firstly, the governmental sector including MoH facilities, which are funded federally by the Ministry of Finance (MoF) [19] and local health authority facilities, i.e. DHA, Abu Dhabi Health Services (SEHA) [20], the operational arm for HAAD, military, police and oil industry facilities. The second major provider of health services is the private sector, whose participation has increased over the last few years. For instance, the public sector operates most major hospitals, while international service providers such as Cleveland Clinic [21] and Johns Hopkins manage a number of Abu Dhabi's institutions. The free medical zones, e.g. Dubai Health Care City, constitute another minor provider of services.

The UAE MoH is an active member in all GCC activities that are managed by the Executive office in Riyadh. The MoH participates as a permanent member in the GCC central registration, price unification meetings and in GCC group purchase tenders, in addition to its contributions to public health initiatives in managing non-communicable, and communicable disease through national immunization programs and establishment of robust protocols for management of pandemics (e.g. H1N1, Corona, etc.). Importantly, the MoH Quality Control Laboratory (QCL) in the UAE is classified as the reference QCL in the GCC.

Payers for the healthcare system are the government, health insurance providers, employers, employees, and individuals, as well as non-profit organizations.

Healthcare quality and reform are top priority in the UAE's government agenda with the state of Abu Dhabi leading the reform. In addition, the MoH has mandated all health facilities to achieve Joint Commission International (JCI) accreditation. Health insurance has become mandatory in the state of Abu Dhabi since 2008, and population insurance coverage reached 99% in 2012. The DHA in Dubai has paved the way toward universal health coverage via implementing the mandatory health insurance 100% by February

2016. Health insurance coverage in other emirates varies between 50% and 80%. Currently, there are more than 42 health insurance providers in the UAE, with the top five being: Daman (UAE National Health Insurance Company) [22], Oman Insurance, Nextcare Arab Gulf Health Services, Nas-Administration Services, and Abu Dhabi National Insurance Company.

Daman established in September 2006, is the first and largest specialized health insurance company to be formed in the UAE as a public joint-stock company that is 80% owned by the Abu Dhabi Government, with the remaining 20% owned by Munich Re (one of the world's leading reinsurers), plays an important role as both reinsurer and a valuable source for knowledge transfer. It currently provides comprehensive health insurance solutions for both individuals and organizations, and exclusively manages both the Government's healthcare program (Thiqa) for UAE nationals, and the Abu Dhabi Basic Plan for low income expatriates. In 2012, HAAD mandated all health insurance providers to implement a Pharmacy Benefit Management (PBM) program. This aimed to mandate pharmacies in Abu Dhabi to seek automated pre-approval from insurers on prescribed medications using HAAD's dedicated transaction platform for healthcare operators and insurers [16]. This step feeds into efforts to obtain accreditation from the Utilization Review Accreditation Commission (URAC) for all health insurers to assure quality services as per international standards.

The implementation of the new Health Information System (HIS) within MoH institution, named "Wareed" is an additional key development in the MoH. The system works to connect patients' data within healthcare facilities including the internal and external departments, radiology, laboratory, pharmacy, surgery, emergency wards, registration, and appointments.

Health technology assessments and economic evaluations are known as the fourth hurdle (after efficacy, safety, and quality) with regard to patient access to new therapies. The incorporation of health economic evidence in optimization of healthcare resources is limited in Middle Eastern countries today. However, there is interest in the UAE and a few other countries to implement economic evaluation formally in the reimbursement system. The aim is to optimize the use of healthcare resources in the future, through implementing Health Information Systems, which will help define, measure and optimize specific healthcare-related outcomes. This step is crucial if the health authorities aim to move into a systematic Health Technology Assessment (HTA) framework.

The Executive Board of the Health Ministers for Arab GCC

The Health Ministers' Council (HMC) for the Cooperation Council States is a regional technical specialized organization established in 1976 with restricted membership. It enjoys juridical identity, and administrative and financial independence. It works to coordinate between the GCC States in the fields of health, and join common world efforts for better achievement of health, based on principles of promotion of cooperation and coordination between the Member States in the preventive, curative, and rehabilitation fields. Specifically, it works to unify and set priorities including adopting common executive programs in Gulf States, such as family health, environmental health, health planning, improving health system performance, quality assurance, primary healthcare, health education, involvement in field surveys and research, procurement of safe and efficient pharmaceutical products and hospital sundries and equipment. Assurance of quality at affordable prices is mainly achieved through the central Group Purchase program and Gulf central registration of pharmaceutical companies and products. The GCC Group Purchasing (GCC-GP) program and central drug registration are examples of powerful activities that impact the pharmaceutical sector in the GCC.

In the Arab Gulf States, strong dominance of governments as main purchasers of drugs through tenders was very common in the past. However, expansion of the private sector has led to an increased market uptake of medicines for diabetes, oncology, and cardiovascular disease [23]. The expansion of the private sector is tightly related to the expansion of high-class private clinics and hospitals on the one hand, and the introduction of mandatory insurance, which have consequently, led to the well-off local population commonly seeking treatment abroad to stay in the region for treatment.

The GCC states have GDPs *per capita* US$ 19,310-97,519 in 2014 [24]. However, the Gulf States spend [25] a much smaller share of their GDP (about 2-4%) on healthcare [26]. This variance could be explained by the fact that in the Gulf countries, the majority of the population is relatively young expatriates, who consume less healthcare services than elderly populations.

The pharmaceutical market in the Arab Gulf States grows at approximately 10% per year in 2006 [27], as per Alpen Capital report, the size of the pharmaceutical industry reached US$ 8.5 billion by the end of 2012, compared to US$ 7.7 billion in 2011. Saudi Arabia produces 59.4% of medicines in the region, followed by 18% in UAE, 9.2% in Kuwait, 5.6% in Oman, 4.5% in Qatar, and finally 3.1% in Bahrain. In addition, the value of the GCC pharmaceutical and healthcare market is expected to triple from US$ 46 billion in early 2012 to an estimated US$ 133 billion in 2018 [28]. The largest figures of *per capita* spending on pharmaceuticals in ME were seen in the UAE, Lebanon, Kuwait, and Qatar in 2008 [11].

Kingdom of Saudi Arabia (KSA)

Healthcare in the Kingdom of Saudi Arabia is mainly provided by the governmental sectors, namely the Ministry of Health (MoH), National Guard Health Affairs, Ministry of Defense, Ministry of Interior and Ministry of Higher Education (through university hospitals), as well as several private sector hospitals.

The MoH also undertakes the overall supervision and follow-up of healthcare-related activities carried out by the private sector. The Minister of Health chairs the health services council. The primary objective of Saudi social development strategy is to provide high standard health services to the general public.

Saudi nationals and residents currently have access to over 400 hospitals, 2,075 healthcare centers, and 850 private clinics. Yet there is a need for expansion in private healthcare because of population growth. Increasing prevalence of obesity, diabetes, cardiovascular diseases, and cancer will create a tremendous demand for more healthcare services [29].

The Saudi population exceeded 28.8 million in 2013. Life expectancy at birth for male/female in 2013 was 74/78. The top four causes of death have been reported as: ischemic heart disease (21.7%), stroke (16%), lower respiratory tract infections (6.3%), and road injury (5.8%) [30].

The Gross Domestic Product of KSA is around US$ 434 billion. Healthcare expenditures account for approximately 4.3% of the GDP. For 2010, the government allocated SR 61.2 billion (US$ 16.31 billion) toward health and social affairs, a 17% increase from the previous year. Total annual pharmaceuticals expenditure increased from US$ 2.65 billion in 2008 to approximately US$ 3.7 billion in year 2013 [29]. The continued government appropriations to the healthcare sector have undoubtedly stimulated the pharmaceutical business environment over the years.

Jordan

Jordan is a small upper-middle income country with limited natural resources. Social security, gender equity and education are rights for all Jordanians [31]. The total population is 7.3 million, total expenditure on health *per capita* is US$ 761 and total expenditure on health share of GDP is 7.2%. Jordan's performance in terms of life expectancy for male/female at birth in 2013 was 72/76. The top four leading causes of death reported in the country in 2012 were Ischemic heart disease (16.8%), stroke (10.7%), diabetes mellitus (6.7%), and road injury (5.5%) [32].

The healthcare system in Jordan includes public and private participation in addition to the Royal Medical Services (RMS) and University Hospitals. The Ministry of Health is responsible for primary preventive healthcare and hospital services. Healthcare services for the armed forces are administered by the Royal Medical Services. In 2013, there were 103 listed hospitals in Jordan, equating to 12,060 hospital beds (18 hospital beds per 10,000 people) [33], with a third of these being in private sector facilities. While the private sector is heavily concentrated in the Amman region, there are some private facilities in other areas in the country. The majority of general practitioners' clinics are private practices. Approximately 87% of the population is insured. The Jordanian Food and Drug Administration (JFDA) is one of the well-established regulating authorities in the region, and is in charge of regulating pharmaceuticals and setting drug prices for sale in community pharmacies and private hospitals in the country [34].

Egypt

Egypt is a lower-middle income country, with a total population of more than 82 million residing in 28 governorates. The healthcare system is fragmented with multiple sources of financing and providers. There are 1969 private and governmental hospitals and 5034 primary healthcare units. Life expectancy at birth for male/female in 2013 was 69/74 [35]. The top four leading causes of death reported in the country in 2012 were ischemic heart disease (21%), stroke (13%), cirrhosis of the liver (8%), and hypertensive heart disease (4%) [35].

The financing sources include government spending that comes from direct tax revenues, out-of-pocket spending, premium payments by households for insurance, employers, and donor assistance from charity organizations [36].

Healthcare services are provided through public sector entities, mainly the Ministry of Health and Population (MOHP) and the Health Insurance Organization (HIO), other ministries and public sector entities such as the Curative Care Organization, teaching hospitals and institutes, and nonprofit non-governmental organizations (NGOs), all in addition to private insurance plans (Egycare). The MOHP owns and operates a large network of hospitals and outpatient facilities. Each public entity runs its own facilities following MOHP regulations while the private sectors have their own set of regulations and standards.

Health spending is 61.4 billion Egyptian pounds (LE) (US$ 7.84 billion), total expenditure on health as a percentage of GDP is 5.1% (2013) [35], while spending on pharmaceuticals accounts for 34% of the total healthcare spending in the country. Although 55% of the population is insured by the HIO as of 2008, the out of pocket spending has increased from 51% to 72% in the past two decades [36].

Lebanon

Lebanon is a small upper-middle income country with a total population of about 4.8 million (2013); the life expectancy at birth for male/female in 2013 was 78/82. In the year 2013, the total expenditure on health *per capita* was US$ 1092 and the total expenditure on health share of GDP was 7.2% [37]. The top four leading causes of death reported in the country in 2012 were ischemic heart disease (31%), stroke (9%), road injury (4%), and diabetes mellitus (4%) [37].

The Ministry of Public Health (MoPH) is the main health regulator and public healthcare provider in the country, it also determines the price of pharmaceutical products in Lebanon [38]. Medical services are dominated by the private sector, which is responsible for 90% of healthcare provision. The government subsidizes private medical bills. According to the World Health Organization (WHO), this has resulted in an oversupply of beds and specialized doctors, but an undersupply of nurses [39]. In fact, the Lebanese primary healthcare system is perceived to be failing to meet its full potential, and the WHO estimates that only 8% of the population benefit from government primary care. Part of the responsibility for this lies with the public. As it is traditional for patients who need treatment to seek advice from specialists, rather than visiting their family doctor [40].

6.4 Pathways of Market Access

The approval process of new drugs to get marketing authorization or license is a regulatory process that involves the assessment of the new drug's safety, efficacy, and quality;

most countries have a national medicine agency responsible for authorizing new pharmaceuticals for marketing and sale.

The registration process of pharmaceutical products in Middle Eastern countries requires a company's registration (including documentation for each manufacturing site and all relevant company subsidiaries), in addition to individual product applications. In some countries, company registration could be applied in parallel to product registration; however, as there are no limits on the approval time for company registration, co-applying may delay product registration. There is also a requirement for a certificate of pharmaceutical product (CPP) at the time marketing authorization is sought; this is usually issued by health authorities on behalf of the manufacturer, the customer in manufacturing country.

In the GCC, under the coordination of the Gulf Committee for Drug Central registration, Gulf countries are harmonizing the marketing application process within their countries. Dossiers are prepared to rigorous standard, mostly typical to the review system of Saudi Arabia [41].

Pricing of pharmaceuticals is complex and is influenced by a number of factors. The complexity of pharmaceutical pricing is a result of the large expenses associated with pharmaceutical research and development. The investment in drug development is a sunk cost at the time the product is launched and drug prices are negotiated [42]. Patent Protection is one of the conventions in pharmaceutical marketing aiming at providing incentives for research and development but also for controlling society's cost of drug treatment.

In Middle Eastern countries, price fixation is generally required for all prescription and some over-the-counter products. A certificate of pricing decision is usually required for each product and it includes information about, among other things, the wholesale price in the country of origin and the registered price in neighboring countries, if available, or in a basket of selected countries (reference-based pricing) [43].

In recent years, GCC members have attempted to align their drug pricing policies with the approval of unified pricing mechanisms and the submission of joint tenders for both public and private sectors [44]. While drug supply in the GCC region has traditionally taken place through the established public healthcare systems, the private sector market is growing rapidly. This is mainly due to evolving compulsory private health insurance requirements for non-nationals. Public sector drug procurement is carried out through closed international tenders, GCC bulk procurement and direct purchasing.

In the Gulf countries, pricing pharmaceuticals, reimbursement negotiations are often based on reference pricing and the basis for inclusion of drugs on national formularies is generally safety, quality and efficacy, but not cost-effectiveness.

Health economics, in particular economic evaluation, has emerged as a method to evaluate the trade-off between the costs and benefits of new drug therapies by those making decisions on reimbursement and market access. Currently, health economic evaluation seems to be limited in the Middle Eastern countries. With the increased introduction of expensive treatments, it is likely that this will become an increasingly important method to establish priorities in healthcare in the region. The International Society of Pharmacoeconomics and Outcomes Research (ISPOR) focuses on emerging regions to facilitate the interchange of scientific knowledge in health economics and outcomes research. In the ME, several countries established a local ISPOR chapter which led to the formulation of the ISPOR Arabic Network. The ISPOR Arabic Network provides a forum to identify important topics for collaborative research and health policy initiatives.

Several senior researchers from the ISPOR Arabic Network joined a pioneer collaborative health policy research initiative to achieve three main objectives. First, to document the extent to which External Price Referencing (EPR) was used in seven ME countries, including Egypt, Jordan, Kuwait, Lebanon, Saudi Arabia, Qatar and the UAE [45]. Second, to assess whether pharmaceutical EPR resulted in narrower price corridor for patented pharmaceuticals compared to non-pharmaceutical services not subjected to EPR. The third objective was to analyze factors influencing pricing of original pharmaceuticals. The study was recently published under the title "Implications of External Price Referencing (EPR) of pharmaceuticals in Middle East countries" and described the pricing system in the UAE, Kuwait, Saudi Arabia, Lebanon, Jordan and Egypt [45]. The study indicated that EPR resulted in a narrower price corridor for innovative pharmaceuticals than outpatient and hospital services. Low income countries could be referenced by higher income countries since the GDP had limited influence on public prices of pharmaceuticals. However, EPR was found to possibly limit timely patient access to new medicines. The survey showed that the use of EPR in the UAE was rational in terms of using mean, median, and lowest price. The study concluded that more research is needed in the ME region to understand the implications of EPR and develop solutions to prevent its negative consequences. Study results are shown in Table 3.

	UAE	Kuwait	Saudi Arabia	Lebanon	Jordan	Egypt
N. referenced countries	31 (including low income countries)	1 (country of origin)	29 (including low income countries)	14 (MENA and European countries)	16 (including low income countries)	35 (including low income countries)
Pricing rule	No strict rule	-	Lowest price	Median price	Median price of at least 4 countries	Lowest price
Referenced by other MENA countries	Egypt, Lebanon, Saudi Arabia	Egypt, UAE, Saudi Arabia	Egypt, Jordan, UAE, Lebanon	Egypt, Saudi Arabia, UAE	Egypt, Saudi Arabia, UAE	Saudi Arabia, Jordan, UAE, Lebanon

Table 3. Survey result for pharmaceuticals External Price Referencing in Middle East countries

MENA = Middle East and North Africa region; UAE = United Arab Emirates

The United Arab Emirates (UAE)

The Ministry of Health is the governing authority responsible for unifying UAE health policies, developing comprehensive nationwide health services and ensuring that healthcare remains accessible across the country. The MoH is the main regulator for the pharmaceutical sector as per the Federal Pharmacy Law 4/1983. Accordingly, the MoH regulates the drug authorization process, pricing policies, health technologies, medical advertisements, clinical studies, post-marketing safety measures and licensing [15]. Various regulations are applied to the development, manufacture, import, marketing, and proper use of drugs and medical devices [46].

Given that the UAE is a highly regulated yet competitive market, many of the world's largest pharmaceutical companies currently have strong presence in the UAE; the majority are re-locating their regional headquarters to the UAE. Other global industry associations such as the Pharmaceutical Research and Manufacturers of America have their regional MENA and Gulf local working group PhRMAG operating out of Dubai.

There are also a number of local pharmaceutical manufacturing companies that are driving innovation in this sector including Julphar, Global Pharma, Neopharma and several others. Notably, there are more than 60 warehouse stores for pharmaceuticals in the free zones in the UAE.

Many regulatory developments took place during the last decade. These include: the voluntary price reduction initiative, a new pricing system, dollarization, GCC price unification, fast track drug approval, implementing national pharmacovigilance standards, regulating medical advertisements, regulating medical devices, herbals and complementary medicines, and implementing the new submission process for drug registration using Common Technical Dossier (CTD) format. It is expected that the eCTD will go live by the end of 2015.

In the UAE, a government measure to bring public drug prices more in line with those in other GCC states was introduced in 2005, and has led to reduced final average selling prices by 7%; a subsequent price cut lowered selling prices by 11%. In 2008, a new pricing system was implemented to include updating currency exchange rates to the UAE Dirham as per the average exchange rate at the UAE Central Bank; the changes affected profit margin for both local agents and pharmacy. The cost containment policies support the government's desire to find a balance between affordable healthcare and international obligations to sustain patent and product quality standards [47].

In 2010, researchers and officials from the MoH conducted a study on medicine price comparisons since there was a public debate published in the media on medicines' prices in the UAE being higher than other GCC countries [48]. The study aimed to compare Cost, Insurance and Freight (CIF) prices in the UAE for selected registered drugs (brands) used in treating chronic diseases with those in other countries. The results demonstrated that the UAE CIF prices were generally higher than Saudi or Jordanian CIF prices for the same product and from the same sources. About 40-50% of the products had very high price differences, with UAE CIF prices being 50-100% higher. The final recommendation was to reduce the CIF price and to use the US dollar as the CIF importing currency (similar to the

GCC-SGH tenders). Both recommendations were in line with the GCC supreme decision for CIF unification and dollarization [48]. As a result, five price reduction initiatives/waves took place on a voluntary basis in collaboration with the industry from 2011 to 2015 [49], while the sixth initiative has just been announced and the effective date is 1st

Initiatives	Year
1st pricing system: total margin = 70% of CIF price (27.5% local agent and 42.5% pharmacy)	1985
2nd pricing system: total margin = 55% of CIF price (25% local agent and 30% pharmacy)	2004
3rd pricing system: total margin = 44% of CIF price (20% local agent and 24% pharmacy)	2005
4th pricing system: total margin range from CIF price = 33-44% related to the currency and medicines use Local agent markup = 10-15% for euro; 20% other currencies Pharmacy profit = 18-24% from CIF price	2008
Price comparison study (MoH study)	2010
Price reduction initiative, waves 1 and 2 565 innovative drugs (reduction between 5% and 55%) 115 drugs (reduction between 5% and 35%)	2011
New pricing criteria implemented Dollarization for CIF and total margin from CIF price = 35-43% Local agent markup = 15% from CIF price Pharmacy profit = 20-28% from CIF price	2013
Price reduction initiative, wave 3 6,619 medicines price reduced between 1% and 40%	2013
GCC price harmonization: dollarization and CIF unification 2,432 medicines been unified/reduced between 5% and 60% The work ongoing for other innovative and generic drugs	2014
MENA External Price Referencing (EPR) Survey, published recently [45]	2014
Price reduction initiative, wave 4 192 innovative drugs; reduction between 1% and 83%	2014
Price reduction initiative, wave 5 [50] 280 innovative medicines reduction of prices between 6% and 55%	2015
Price reduction initiative, wave 6 188 innovative medicines to be reduced 1% and 50% was implemented in January 2016	2016
The seventh price reduction initiative been announced for 653 innovative medicine and planned to be implemented by 1st September 2016	2016

Table 4. Pricing history and milestones, Ministry of Health, United Arab Emirates
CIF = Cost, Insurance and Freight (UAE); MENA = Middle East and North Africa region; MoH = Ministry of Health

---

Box 1. New pricing system in the United Arab Emirates (effective date 6ᵗʰ June 2013)

1. Cost, Insurance and Freight (CIF) prices for all imported medicines are in US$ (as per medicine category).
2. New profit margins:
   - total margin = 35-43% from CIF price to retail price/public price;
   - local agent profit margin = 15% of CIF/11% of WholeSale Price(WSP);
   - pharmacy profit margins = 17-24% of WSP/20-28% from CIF (the ex-factory price in AED, the currency used in the United Arab Emirates, for local companies will substitute for the CIF import price AED).
3. Medicines are categorized in 3 categories as per CIF price in AED.

A	B	C
CIF ≤ 250 AED	CIF > 250 to 500 AED	CIF > 500 AED
Pharmacy margin = 24% (28% of CIF)	Pharmacy margin = 20% (24% of CIF)	Pharmacy margin = 17% (20% of CIF)

January 2016. Pricing history in the UAE and associated milestones are described in Table 4.

In June 2013, a new pricing system was applied in the UAE, where dollarization is standardized. Five waves of price reductions took place to achieve unifications with other GCC countries, and a margin adjustment. As mentioned earlier, new pricing criteria were implemented on 6ᵗʰ June 2013. The official imported prices are the CIF prices, which needed to be in US dollars. The local agent margin became 15% of the CIF price for any medicine and the pharmacy profit with segmented margins as per CIF value are now between 17% and 24% of wholesale price. The total margin for both local agents and pharmacies ranges between 35% and 43% of the CIF price. Key changes in the new pricing system are described in Box 1.

At the same time, the GCC CIF unification and dollarization process started in July 2013 leading to a series of meetings to implement the CIF unification in phases, as per drug therapeutic class.

Name	% reduction 2014 prices
Lipitor®	About 9.4%
Augmentin®	Estimated savings using 2014 prices (10,462,000 US$ is the approximate total saving for top 5 brands by value)
Janumet®	
Crestor®	
Nexium®	

Table 5. Price reduction for top 5 branded drugs in 2013

An example of cost savings due to price reduction for the top 5 branded drugs in value as per the IMS drug market report 2013 is presented in Table 5.

The UAE imports about 84% of all its medicines; 16% are manufactured locally [51]. The regulatory culture in the UAE is robust since the government supports intellectual property protection. Fast track approval to accelerate access to innovative drugs such as Bydureon® (exenatide), Gilenya® (fingolimod), Trulicity® (dulaglutide) made the UAE the third fastest country in the world to approve these types of drugs [52].

One of the recent key regulatory developments in the UAE was the implementation of the national pharmacovigilance program in 2009. Currently, the UAE is a member in the Uppsala Monitoring Center (UMC). In addition, the registration process for each registered medicine requires that a mandatory pharmacovigilance risk management plan is submitted with all registration documents.

Other developments in the UAE include banning all health-related advertisements that have not been thoroughly vetted by the MoH. The move is an attempt to protect the public from misleading or false medical promises.

The Executive Board of the Health Ministers for Arab GCC

As mentioned earlier, the GCC central drug registration and the group purchasing program are the main activities that impact the pharmaceutical sector in the GCC, and are managed under the Executive Board of the Health Ministers for Arab GCC. The GCC central drug registration [53] started in 2001 by implementing the ministerial decision of the GCC Conference for Health Ministerial Council session 1/2001 about activating the central registration system which took more than 10 years in study, review and audit. Its main goals [4] are listed in Box 2.

The central registration section established a unified supervisory registration system for the manufactures and their products and highlighted the benefit of sharing supervisory drug laboratories within the GCC member countries. Currently, it works to develop a

---

Box 2. Central registration goals

1. Unify the registration of pharmaceutical companies of the Gulf Cooperation Council (GCC) countries.
2. Unify the regulations and procedures in the registration of pharmaceutical companies and products.
3. Unify the pricing of drugs are marketed in the GCC countries.
4. Promote greater integration and coordination between member states in pharmaceutical sector.
5. Consolidate information and conditions at the drug registration.
6. Ensure the application of good manufacturing practice by manufacturing companies.
7. Monitor medicines quality and promote adverse effect reporting.
8. Promote the rational use and access to safe and effective medication at lowest cost.

---

central drug registration policy, issue GMP regulations and bylaws, and supervise accreditation of quality control reference laboratories.

Recently, the central registration section established a pricing unit to implement CIF price unification and dollarization in the GCC countries based on the supreme council decision in December, 2007. The decision mandated state members to unify CIF export prices of medicines to the GCC countries as per the lowest in the GCC, which are most likely those of KSA, use the US dollars as a formal import currency for all CIF prices (dollarization), and control total mark-up for both local agent and pharmacy to assure that the public price in any GCC country does not exceed 45% of CIF price.

On the other hand, group purchasing, which is managed under the Executive Board of the Health Ministers for Arab GCC, is used extensively as a cost saving method by taking advantage of bulk purchasing power via tender prices. The GCC-GP Program procures jointly for Ministries of Health and other participating health sectors in the GCC, its tenders known as Secretariat General of Health (SGH) tenders. The tender initially started with 32 pharmaceutical products in 1978, with a value of about one million US dollars. Due to the great success of this program, tender items and value increased dramatically; currently there are 16 SGH tenders and the total tender's value equated to US$ 2,999,255,794 in 2014 [4].

In addition to cost savings due to the power of bulk purchasing, there are many advantages to the GCC group purchasing program such as: saving efforts and resources by minimizing administrative and regulatory burdens on the ministries of health; dealing with pre-qualified/certified manufacturers that follow cGMP; and adopting registered/pre-evaluated/technically-accepted health technology. Furthermore, the process is transparent with pre-published general and technical terms and conditions and award criteria

---

Box 3. The GCC group purchase tenders (SGH tenders) in 2014

1. Medicines.
2. Vaccines and sera.
3. Chemicals.
4. Insecticides.
5. Radiopharmaceuticals.
6. Renal dialysis solutions.
7. Hospital sundries.
8. Renal dialysis supplies.
9. Laboratory supplies and blood transfusion services.
10. Rehabilitation supplies (2013 for two years).
11. Orthopedic and spine supplies (2013 for two years).
12. Dental and mouth care supplies.
13. Cardiovascular surgery, interventional cardiology and interventional radiology supplies.
14. Linens and medical uniforms (2013 for two years).
15. ENT (2014 for two years).
16. Ophthalmic supplies (2014 for two years).

Steps	Communication	Timeline	Action by
Tender preparation	Meeting 1		All participating members
Initial quantities	E-communication	3 weeks	All participating members
Announcing tender	Direct/publish	6 weeks	GP Section-Executive office Riyadh-KSA
Open envelopes/ offers	Meeting 2	2 weeks	All participating members
Bid study and selection	Meeting 3	2 weeks	All participating members
Publish primary selection/award	Direct/publish		All participating members
Appeal/complain	Meeting 4	1 weeks	All participating members
Publish final selection	Direct/publish		GPP Section-Executive office Riyadh- KSA
Final quantities	E-communication	Subjective to tender	All participating members
Award notification	Executive office Riyadh-KSA		GPP Section
Purchase orders	Participating states	4 weeks	All participating members
Monitoring-follow up	GPP and all partici-pating members		GPP and all participating members

Table 6. Gulf Cooperation Council-Secretariat General Health (GCC-SGH) tender process
KSA = Kingdom of Saudi Arabia

which include an appeal system. In addition, SGH tenders support the economy and the industry in the GCC by providing 5% and 3% support advantages for products that are manufactured fully or partially respectively in the GCC through promoting innovation and transfer of high technology and under-licensed manufacturing.

Other advantages to SGH tendering include supporting the research fund by deducting 2% of the awarded amount for the welfare of the GCC member states, In addition, to sharing experiences and information about safety, quality for any related problems among countries, institutions, and hospitals, and finally, ensuring continuous supply of drugs, medical supplies all year round through regular successive deliveries. SGH group tender names in 2014 are listed in Box 3, and SGH tender process is presented in Table 6.

Kingdom of Saudi Arabia (KSA)

The Saudi pharmaceutical market is the largest in the Arab region. Pharmaceuticals manufactured locally account for 15%, while imported pharmaceuticals account for 85% [29]. A rapidly growing population is an important market determinant.

The pharmaceutical market in Saudi Arabia is a highly regulated market. The Ministry of Health (MoH) was the main regulatory authority responsible for regulating the pharmaceutical sector in the country. In 2009, the Saudi Food and Drug Authority (SFDA) took over pharmaceutical registration from the MoH. Currently, SFDA is responsible for developing and enforcing a transparent regulatory system for the pharmaceutical sector and is considered a major regulatory agency in KSA [54].

Many factors affect pharmaceutical pricing, including drug therapeutic significance, the prices of similar registered alternative drugs, outcomes of pharmacoeconomics studies, ex-factory price in the country of origin, wholesale price in the country of origin, public price in the country of origin, additional cost to KSA such as: CIF price, export price to countries where the drug is registered, and lastly, prices in official pricing references (when available). Often, the price of the innovative drug is decreased by 20% after the registration of its first generic drug, whereas the first generic drug price is expected to be 35% lower than that of the innovative drug. Further generic drug prices are lowered by 10% for each subsequent drug introduced [55].

Pharmaceutical Companies have the right to appeal against pricing decisions. The price approved by the SFDA is considered to be a ceiling price. Final actual purchasing prices for different healthcare sectors are subject to negotiation, the tendering process and the purchasing power.

Factually, drug registration and pricing do not guarantee the reimbursement by different healthcare sectors such as the National Guard Health Affairs, Ministry of Health, Ministry of Defense, Ministry of Interior, Ministry of Higher Education (university hospitals) and in the health insurance companies [29], as it is subject to their formularies.

Jordan

The Jordanian Food and Drug Administration regulates medicines in Jordan. Pharmaceutical companies submit files to JFDA for registering and pricing new chemical entities (originator brand) [34]. The price for a new chemical entity is determined based on the lowest price resulting from considering the following: CIF price, the public price in the country of origin, the median public price in at least 4 countries from the following reference countries (UK, France, Spain, Italy, Belgium, Greece, Netherlands, Australia, Cyprus, Hungary, Ireland, New Zealand, Portugal, Check, Croatia, and Austria), plus the export price to Saudi Arabia. In the case where the innovative drug is registered only in the country of origin and in 3 countries or less, the drug is priced based on the lowest price resulting from the mean price in these countries. For generics, the price should not exceed 80% of the originator price. Where there is a price reduction in the originator drug, all generics must reduce their prices, except where the price is due to an exchange rate movement or at the request of the originator. Drug prices are usually revised after 2 years of registration. In addition, all prices are reviewed every 5 years upon registration renewal.

The majority of insurance coverage is through public schemes and institutions, such as the military, the United Nation Relief and Works Agency (UNRWA), universities and the Civil health Insurance Program (CIP), which covers government employees. Employer-based schemes and private sector insurance are other options available.

The Jordanian government has extended its national health insurance scheme to cover pregnant women and those aged 60 years and above. The initiative was launched in May 2006, with the issuance of 15,000 medical insurance cards to eligible residents, prior to being rolled out across the country. The scheme is entirely voluntary and if the necessary treatment could not be provided in government hospitals, the patient would be treated at an army-run establishment. The Health Insurance Fund mainly receives funds from the state budget and from fees provided by beneficiaries. In January 2012, Jordan-based Arab Orient Insurance Company entered into an agreement with a French global reinsurance company to launch the biggest medical reinsurance portfolio in Jordan. Recently, in February 2015, the private healthcare provider MedNet Jordan announced it had signed a cooperation agreement with the Royal Medical Services (RMS) facilities and Ministry of Health hospitals to expand their healthcare services to members of MedNet Jordan [33].

Egypt

The Ministry of Health and Population is the decision maker for market authorization and drug reimbursement in the public sector. The MOHP executes the legal and regulatory framework for healthcare interventions and the Health Insurance Act, and overall health policy. It has the responsibility for health system regulation and oversees the Health Insurance Organization, Central Administration for Pharmaceutical Affairs (CAPA), National Organization for Drug Control and Research (NODCAR) and National Organization for Research and Control of Biologicals (NORCB). The three organizations, CAPA, NODCAR, and NORCB constitute the "Egyptian Drug Authority" (EDA). CAPA, being part of the MOHP, has the responsibility for price regulation and decision making regarding prices of drugs available to the public [36,56].

Currently, there are two prices for each drug marketed within the country: the mandated government retail price and the tender price. Pricing decisions are compliant with the pharmaceutical Egyptian price regulations. CAPA reevaluates pricing of drugs every three years and upon request of the drug manufacturers in case of changes in costs, new indications or changed exchange rate by 15%. Additionally, the price of the product may be changed in case of marketing of cheaper equivalent in any country. For branded products, pricing is based on a reference pricing model of 10% less than the lowest referenced country price. Annual price reduction by 2% once the first generic is approved is usually adopted. For generic products, a reduction is applied from the lowest referenced country price by 30% if the product is certified by Food and Drug Administration (FDA), European Medicines Agency (EMA) or Therapeutic Goods Administration (TGA), or the manufacturer is accredited by WHO, or a member in International Council on Harmonisation of technical requirements for registration of pharmaceuticals for human use (ICH). If the product is locally manufactured and licensed by CAPA, a reduction of 40% is applied; while a 60% reduction is applied for products manufactured in another country [36].

The procurement department at MOHP normally conducts needs assessment and informs manufacturers about quantities needed of different drugs. Drug manufacturers submit bids to the Procurement Technical Committee, which reviews all MOHP hospitals and primary care units' needs of medications and makes a determination. The procurement department publishes approved tender drug list. The reimbursement process in Egypt usually covers most drugs in the market.

Stability in drug prices is an important advantage to the current pricing regulations in Egypt. However, this system limits innovation and contains loopholes that allow pharmaceutical companies to circumvent the rules and obtain the highest possible price for their products regardless of their true cost. A gap exists between Health Technology Assessment research and actual reimbursement decision making in Egypt; however, recently, a ministerial decree was passed to the establishment of a Pharmacoeconomic Unit at CAPA [36].

Lebanon

The Ministry of Health determines the price of pharmaceutical products in Lebanon. The price of an imported drug is based on the cost in the country of origin, with the final price being lower than any of the following: the ex-factory price in the country of origin, import prices charged for the same brand in seven countries in the Middle East, the median manufacturers' price in seven European countries, or the import price of similar drugs that are already marketed in Lebanon. Authorities also determine importers' and pharmacists' mark-ups, which are digressive; the higher the price of the drug, the lower the mark-up. Factors used to fix the price of locally-manufactured drugs include the cost of production, the public price of similar products marketed in Lebanon, cost and profit index and the classification of pharmaceutical manufacturing companies. Prices must be registered with the ministry, with data on product price in the currency of the country of origin being required [38].

In June 2010, with the aim of containing healthcare costs, the MoH announced that price cuts of up to 23% were implemented on 118 pharmaceuticals which were mainly for hypertension and cardiovascular disease. The decision follows the more extensive price reductions of around 1,000 drugs in 2004 and 2005. In June 2014, the MoH minister issued an amended pharmaceutical bill where the price of high-cost drugs would be reduced by between 10% and 17%. Other recent developments include reducing the prices of 60 generic and 30 branded drugs in March 2015. In addition, a new legislation requiring pharmaceutical companies to report any decrease in price in any of the referenced countries has been implemented recently.

Despite medicines' prices in Lebanon being among the lowest in the ME due to its reference pricing legislation, reducing healthcare costs in Lebanon would be key to maximizing healthcare coverage.

The Ministry of Public Health is responsible for regulating and procuring 10% of the drugs purchased in Lebanon. This provides some biopharmaceutical drugs free of charge for patients suffering from cancer, multiple sclerosis, mental illness and other chronic conditions covering around 12,000 patients at this time. Around 40% of the Lebanese population has no form of health insurance coverage. The remaining 60% are insured either through public or private insurance. There are two drug reimbursement institutions in Lebanon, the National Social Security Fund (NSSF) and the Cooperative of Civil Servants (CCS). The NSSF reimburses 80% of the drug healthcare bill with 20% copay and covers private sector employees, while the CCS reimburses 75% of the drug bill with 25% copay and covers public sector employees. However, only 20% of medicines consumed in the country are thought to be reimbursed through either of the two schemes. According to official figures, some 140,000 low-income patients are also covered through the Young Men's Christian Association (YMCA) [40].

Seemingly, a reimbursement system would be useful in the public planning of healthcare spending, and would make more informed decisions on the uptake of health technologies. Efforts to improve drug access, coupled with gradual economic development and increased political stability, should help improve the situation [38].

6.5 Mapping and Structure of Decision Makers

Health outcomes research studies the end results of medical care, the effect of the healthcare process on the health and well-being of patients and populations [57]. This type of research has been increasingly conducted in a range of medical and therapeutic areas, especially high public concern areas, studying the unmet medical needs and current treatment patterns as new clinical innovations and new drugs are developed. An economic evaluation is "the comparative analysis of alternative courses of action in terms of both their costs and their consequences" [58]. Outcomes research can provide baseline data for cost-effectiveness analyses to be conducted. Health Economic evaluations conducted to inform healthcare resource allocation in the Middle Eastern countries are limited. The high prevalence rates and costs associated with treatment of conditions of public concern such as Type 2 Diabetes Mellitus (T2DM) make these types of analyses much needed. With the introduction of new technologies, especially high-cost treatments, it is likely that economic evaluation will become an increasingly important method to make priorities in healthcare in the region, to optimize care and plan the provision of coverage of healthcare for the population.

Currently, there is a growing interest in Health Technology Assessment (HTA) and economic evaluation among healthcare providers and health insurance companies within the GCC countries. In the UAE, the use of pharmacoeconomic and HTA assessments as decision making tools in formulary inclusion and reimbursement are paving their way within HAAD and DHA institutions. Retrospective observational chart reviews funded by research funds from pharmaceutical companies working in close collaboration with academic institutions and the Dubai Health Authority in the areas of T2DM, atrial fibrillation, hepatitis C have been conducted. These highlighted the importance of investigating the unmet medical needs and the cost implications of current practice in the UAE [59].

Challenges and Catalyzers for Market Access

Barriers to the use of economic evaluation in policy decision-making in Middle Eastern countries are existing, and it might simulate those barriers found in Asian countries [60]. Such as barriers related to the production of economic information, topic prioritization, the availability of economic evaluation guidelines, lacking of understanding of economic evaluation, politics and decision context-related barriers, where the recommended solutions are: standardizing economic evaluation methods, publishing economic evaluations, educating stakeholders including decision-makers, health professionals, and the public, making the economic evaluation processes transparent and participatory, and incorporating other health preferences into the decision-making framework such as equity, necessity, and social solidarity.

The United Arab Emirates (UAE)

The aims for the UAE vision 2021 is to place the UAE among the top ten best countries in the world by 2021. Therefore, much effort has been put into achieving this goal [13].

The favorable investment environment, strong Intellectual Property governance, regulations and fast track approval for innovative and life-saving drugs are key drivers that

---

Box 4. Driving factors promoting healthcare and pharmaceutical market in the UAE

- The UAEs competitiveness position that attracts investments in research and biotechnology.
- Growing population in terms of size and life expectancy.
- Health insurance models as the dominant way of health funding.
- Regulatory enhancements.
- Private sector participation growth share.
- Lifestyle-related diseases are highly prevalent in the UAE (diabetes, obesity, hypertension, and osteoporosis).
- UAE being the medical tourism hub in the region: in August 2014, the UAE announced an amended visa policy with new specific options for medical tourists. This amendment is part of the UAE's strategy to develop into a major medical tourism hub over the coming years.
- The market share held by the private healthcare sector has risen significantly in recent years. The growth of private healthcare insurance, patient fees and co-payments has substantially boosted overall health spending.
- Public-Private Partnerships (PPPs) will continue to play an important role in driving growth in the UAE's healthcare sector.
- Dubai successful bid to host the 2020 World Expo, the associated investment in infrastructure will have a positive effect on the healthcare market, raising the UAE's appeal as a tourist destination, bringing benefits to the medical tourism sector in its wake.

---

made the UAE one of the most attractive markets to pharmaceutical manufactures. In fact, the UAE is ranked 12th in the recent Global Competitiveness Report 2014-2015 [14].

The growth in the UAE population, and the matching large scale investments in healthcare services to provide comprehensive care pathways and medical skills and resources in treating the increasing prevalence of diseases such as diabetes, cancer and cardiovascular disease are key catalyzers driving the healthcare sector.

The UAE government is facilitating this catalysis by moving toward mandatory healthcare insurance coverage for the whole population which requires rational market access pathways of medical technologies that enable a balance between effectiveness and cost, but without delaying registration and access by patients.

Another factor driving the healthcare system and the pharmaceutical market in the UAE is medical tourism; the UAE is becoming a major hub in the region.

Collaboration between regulators, providers, payers, academia and the industry along with patient groups is required to carry out comprehensive outcomes studies that evaluate and measure the driving factors in the pharmaceutical sector and healthcare market in the UAE to improve standards and the regulatory environment. Examples for catalyzers and driving factors that promote the healthcare and pharmaceutical market in the UAE are listed in Box 4.

Optimal market access indicates the importance of minimizing the time for approval of new drugs (to improve patient accessibility), without reducing the quality of the evaluation and the decision process. In achieving this aim, a number of challenges need to be overcome. These are related to the approval times, formulary inclusion, new insurance

---

Box 5. Key challenges for market access

- Scattered health care data among healthcare providers and payers.
- Insufficient communications and collaboration between academia and key stakeholders.
- Insufficient number of national experts and professionals.
- Need to build capacity/qualified and skilled human resources, National HTA Agency.
- Need to include pharmacoeconomics, health economics, and Health Technology Assessments (HTAs) in medicine, pharmacy, health science and nursing curricula.
- Underdeveloped patient advocacy groups and lack of collaboration between stakeholders with such groups and consumer association.
- Lack of independent research to assess and evaluate the key attributes and barriers in pharmacy and healthcare sector, one of the challenges related to the willingness for healthcare institutions to share data and collaborate with the pharmaceutical industry on research projects to inform decision making.
- Lack of pharmacoeconomic guidelines, HTA and outcomes research.
- Insufficient clinical and economic support tools that help decision makers.
- Need for unique identity national drug code for each medicines/product line (data-matrix).

and reimbursement systems and the need to accelerate the diffusion of knowledge in research.

To assess new technologies, a systematic approach with clear and transparent guidelines should be implemented. The current assessment for reimbursement rarely includes a systematic approach. Furthermore, cost-effectiveness analysis is sometimes limited to the review of published foreign evaluations with little localization of international cost-effectiveness models and integration of country-level epidemiological data. The availability of data, and use of research to inform decision making, is still lacking. A number of projects have been conducted for use in decision making, but they are at an early stage, further capability building and awareness of definition of value are strategically needed. Key challenges are listed in Box 5.

In the short term, local cost-effectiveness evaluations will have limited use if performed by the technology producer without validating the assumptions and modeling scenarios through discussions with payers.

Mutual work is required from both the manufacturer as well as the payer, the lack of expertise in health economics within the region, mainly from the payer side is very limiting, making this an area for improvement in the UAE and other ME countries.

It is crucial for health authorities to develop guidelines and frameworks for health economic evaluation if they aim to make evidence based reimbursement decisions in the future. Without guidelines, pharmaceutical companies will not be able to provide the necessary data to help the authorities make choices and decide how to allocate their resources effectively and efficiently.

Technology producers could use their HTA submissions in established HTA markets to discuss with local payers the modeling process and assumptions used and cooperate with them on introducing necessary adaptations to the local contexts.

Challenges: Industry Perspectives

There is a number of challenges associated with the regulatory, registration, pricing, and reimbursement of innovative drugs. Upon interviewing industry stakeholders, some of the risks and challenges were discussed, and are highlighted in this section.

Several improvements to the process of registration are reflected through streamlined processes and fast track submissions for innovative and life-saving drugs. However, there are still some challenges that pharmaceutical companies face when seeking registration of innovative products. For example, when filing for registration in the UAE, pharmaceutical companies are required to report the price of the new product in the country of origin. There are cases where the pharmaceutical companies seek early access for certain innovative products even before a price is published in the country of origin. Pricing rules for such cases are not clear and as a result, companies may be reluctant to fast track a product if it has not been registered and priced in the country of origin. Other concerns are related to the pressure exerted by health authorities on prices of innovative drugs. The cost of drug development has risen substantially in recent years, it can be close to about one billion dollars with several years of research and development [61]. Enforcing price reductions for innovative products may de-incentivize the innovation and investment in research and development sought at the local level which is against anticipation of several GCC countries to become a hub for research and development in the Middle East.

Other challenges could be associated with the impact of reference pricing in the Middle East on access to innovation where different regions in the area represent a range of low to medium to high income countries. There are always concerns that EPR lead to delays in access to medicine, especially in countries where the price is expected to be among the lowest [62]. The industry in general is not in favor of international reference pricing as it hinders the ability of pharmaceutical companies to adjust their prices based on market conditions and the value of the product at the national level. Tier and dynamic pricing models based on the value of the product allow pharmaceutical companies to adjust their prices based on several factors including the affordability of different populations, resulting in a wider access to affordable medicine.

Finally there is still some degree of reluctance to collaborate with the pharmaceutical industry on research, especially outcomes-based research. Research collaboration is an important catalyzer to optimizing market access, and diffusing scientific knowledge among different stakeholders. Although there are some good examples in this field, including retrospective observational chart review studies which have been conducted in the UAE and other countries in the Middle East [59], there are still many opportunities for collaboration to optimize the delivery and outcomes of healthcare.

6.7 Examples from Market Access Strategies

Outcomes research can form baseline data for future improvements. And when data were made available, cost-effectiveness analyses are conducted. So far, cost analyses and cost-effectiveness analyses are at an early stage of development for the Middle East region; however with high prevalence rates and high costs associated with treatment of T2DM, treatment patterns and outcomes should be evaluated in order to optimize diabetic care, and plan the provision of coverage of healthcare for the population, which is manifested with insurance coverage and systems.

The following examples have been implemented in the UAE and other neighboring ME markets including:

Non Communicable Disease (NCD) – Patient Assistance Programs – Oncology, Differential Pricing Strategy

Cost sharing is an example for successful strategies that promote access to high cost innovative medicines for patients under basic health insurance plans or those who do not have insurance at all, through patient assistance programs that were facilitated by non-profit, patient support agencies, in collaboration with pharmaceutical companies and charities, under supervision of MOH. In such collaborations, the pharmaceutical company provides 30-70% of the annual treatment course free of charge while the patient and/or the charity organization covers the rest of the treatment course. This program started in the ME in 2011-2012. "Musanda Patient Assistance Program" is an example for program; it was implemented in the UAE in 2013, as partial payment program designed to improve access to innovative drug to treat macular degeneration, then been expanded to include the first oral drug for multiple sclerosis, for patients who pay out-of-pocket for their treatment in the UAE. Patients pay only what they can afford based on personalized financial assessment results and receive the remainder of the treatment free. It has since been expanded later on to include several oncology products [63].

Non Communicable Disease – Diabetes, Public Private Partnership Aimed at Capacity Building Through an Integrated Educational Platform

Local Initiative

In the countries of the Eastern Mediterranean Region, the prevalence of diabetes ranges between 3.5 and 25.0 percent of the population [64]. The United Arab Emirates is one of the highest prevalence rates of diabetes and as per recent report by the International Diabetes Federation Atlas is estimated at 19% of the population [65], while the prevalence as per 1998-2000 data was 24%, of which is T2DM at more than 90% [66].

A first class experience of the DHA, with the objective of meeting the key performance indicators (KPI) of the 2021 vision of the Ministry of Health to reduce the prevalence of diabetes was trialed through a structured educational program. Details were published at the DHA portal with all related links [67-71].

Other Local Initiatives

MENA Leadership Forum Dubai

As part of ongoing efforts to address the global diabetes epidemic, the World Diabetes Foundation (WDF) in partnership with the Executive Board, Health Ministers' Council for Gulf Cooperation Council States, the World Bank Group MENA Region and the UAE Ministry of Health, have co-hosted the MENA Diabetes Leadership Forum in Dubai as part of company Changing Diabetes® Leadership Initiative that demonstrates its commitment to facilitating a worldwide response to the escalating prevalence of diabetes in every country. The forum helped to gather about 700 participants from 22 countries and territories in the MENA region representing governments, healthcare professionals and patient associations, research and academic institutes, think tanks, business and media. Topics addressed include diabetes prevention and treatment, wellness and healthy lifestyles, with the purpose of sharing knowledge and exploring a regional action plan to reverse the trend in diabetes.

Changing Diabetes World Tour

Changing Diabetes World Tour is a mobile diabetes screening initiative organized by International Pharmaceutical Company and Steno Diabetes Centre under the patronage and support of the UAE Ministry of Health. The objective of the Changing Diabetes® World Tour is to help identify people who have diabetes or are at high risk of developing diabetes without knowing it. Visitors are offered the following tests: blood glucose reference test (HbA1c), blood pressure, hip and waist circumference, Body Mass Index (BMI) and total cholesterol.

Regional Initiatives

Action on Diabetes in Qatar:

The "Action on Diabetes" program is a unique Public-Private Partnership established in 2011 between the pharmaceutical industry, Maersk Oil and the local healthcare authorities in Qatar (Supreme Council of Health, Hamad Medical Corporation, Primary Healthcare Corporation and Qatar Diabetes Association) to help Qatari Healthcare Authorities tackle the diabetes problem in the country by: supporting local diabetes research and rolling out the 1st National Diabetes Registry, conducting awareness campaigns for people living with diabetes and offering education to healthcare professionals, and screening more than 30,000 people for diabetes.

"Action on Diabetes" has run more than 20 projects over the last 3 years including the participation as a full partner with the "National Diabetes Commission" which is formed by a ministerial decree to devise the "National Diabetes Strategy" for Qatar.

National Diabetes Centre (NDC) in Saudi:

NDC is a joint-effort between Gulf and the Saudi Society for Family and Community Medicine. The centre provides diabetes education courses to pharmacists, nurses and doctors, nutrition specialists and dieticians from all over KSA and nurses from other Gulf countries. Key speakers are invited from various institutions in KSA.

Access to Innovation – 1st Oral Multiple Sclerosis Therapy Regulatory Fast Track Introduction

The case of fingolimod (Gilenya®) was unique in the UAE since it was the first oral therapy for a serious disease, Multiple Sclerosis (MS). In an interview with Head of Market Access MENA, he explained that there was a unique opportunity to bring this innovative therapy to the UAE market as early as possible so that MS patients could benefit from it. The Market Authorization Holder (MAH) worked diligently with the UAE MoH to bring it to the market. In this fashion, the UAE was the first in the Middle East and the third country in the world (after the United States and Russia) to have it approved. The MoH gave this innovative drug conditional approval after one week of submission (submission 5th October 2010, approval 12th October 2010), and accepted the file with commitments from Market Authorization Holder to submit all missing documents (CPP, etc.)

shortly after the product was approved in the country of origin (Switzerland). Close collaboration between the company and the MoH allowed patients to have early access to this life-saving therapy. This speaks to the willingness to consider non-traditional pathways to bring products to patients in the UAE early on for diseases with high unmet medical needs in the UAE.

Access to Unmet Need – Curative Hepatitis C Virus (HCV) Therapies

Example from Egypt

Hepatitis C is a serious infection commonly encountered in Egypt. The MOHP is making efforts to lower the prevalence of the disease by raising awareness and supporting access to HCV treatment. Currently, there are three approved products Directly Acting Antivirals (DAAs) for the treatment of HCV in Egypt; Sofosbuvir (Sovaldi®), Simeprevir (Olysio®), and Daclatasvir (Clatazev®). The fix dose combination of sofosbuvir and ledipasvir (Harvoni®) will be available by the end of year 2015. The MOHP has signed an agreement with the Market Authorization Holder of sofosbuvir (Sovaldi®) to offer a discount in the value of 99% of the drug's original price [72], when sofosbuvir is produced locally. A local factory to produce sofosbuvir (Sovaldi®) locally was established in May 2015.

Non Communicable Disease – Diabetes, Payer Partnership – Disease Management Program

Example from the UAE: i-ACT

One of the major challenges in market access strategies in the Middle East is the lack of Real World Data (RWD). In respect to pricing and market access strategy, RWD may support claims for premium price and development of innovative reimbursement schemes.

Partnership of MAH with payers in the collection of RWD may be a vital option to improve payer understanding of diseases and their management, facilitating pricing and reimbursement (P&R) decisions and providing opportunities for best reward of innovation. Likewise, the emergence of new Health Technologies (HT) with questions in cost-effectiveness, may increase the need for RWD to support payers' understanding of the economic and clinical values of new HT. Pharmaceutical and medical device companies must work with payers to move toward local data generation.

Disease management programs are designed to improve the health of persons with chronic conditions and reduce associated costs from avoidable complications by identifying and treating chronic conditions more quickly and effectively [73]. In the Middle East, disease management programs are in the early stages with only a few attempts to implement such programs through partnership between payers and pharmaceutical companies. In 2011, international health insurance company with LifeScan launched a 12-month management program that aimed to help patients with diabetes in the Gulf countries manage their condition.

The i-Act is a comprehensive diabetes management program designed to help people with diabetes comply with the treatment and lifestyle changes necessary to avoid complications that can lead to serious health consequences. The program provides education, free access to medical specialists, diabetes educators and a blood glucose testing kit for each patient enrolled in the program. The program is complimentary and is open to all its health insurance cardholders and their dependents who are diagnosed with the condition. Enrolling in the program is on a voluntary and confidential basis. In the Middle East, a region with high prevalence of diabetes, most of health plans exclude coverage of glucometer strips. Most of health insurance plans exclude miscellaneous healthcare services or apply high co-payments against such services. This program is pioneer in terms of new healthcare coverage and the vision for patient's education. Currently, more than 20,000 diabetic patients have the opportunity to benefits from the i-Act program.

6.8 Look up for the Near Future

The future expansion of access to medicines in the Middle-East and in particular the UAE will depend on:
1. the establishment of public private partnerships;
2. availability of data;
3. implementation of pharmacoeconomic guidelines; and
4. integration of best available evidence in clinical practice.

The implementation of compulsory health insurance in the UAE will be a key driver for the establishment of Public-Private Partnerships. The examples above have illustrated how partnerships between the Ministry of Health, health authorities and private sector stakeholders can be effective in establishing collaboration around priority disease areas, e.g. diabetes. In the future Public-Private Partnerships will enable regulators and pharmaceutical companies to align objectives, develop focused plans that integrate and share resources, and reduce the burden of disease through targeted interventions.

To strengthen decision-making in the future, good data will be needed particularly on cost variables and resource utilization rates in both public and private health facilities. These inputs are essential for conducting burden of illness studies and determining the economic value of current and new medicines. Comprehensive cost data covering outpatient and inpatient services will enable researchers and regulators to make resource allocation decisions and prioritize the introduction of health technologies including new medicines and medical devices.

The development and implementation of pharmacoeconomic guidelines in the UAE will elevate the role and application of scientific standards for the pharmacoeconomic evaluation of medicines and pharmaceutical programs. Pharmacoeconomics is used in price-setting decisions, designing formularies, and guiding reimbursement policy by regulators, pharmaceutical companies, health insurance firms, academic institutions and health consultants. The results of pharmacoeconomic studies have far-reaching implications for patient access to medicines. Pharmacoeconomic guidelines will standardize the application of pharmacoeconomic methods; clarify the use of study perspectives, discount rates, cost-effectiveness thresholds; and outline the structure of pharmacoeconomic submissions and the conditions for mandatory inclusion in regulatory approval processes.

The rapid expansion of the healthcare system in the UAE, a highly diverse and predominantly internationally-trained health work force, growth in the number and type of private providers, and the delivery of compulsory health insurance benefits through private health insurance companies are all factors that strengthen the need for evidence-based clinical practice guidelines. In the future the guidelines will integrate the best available evidence and suggest the quantity and quality of health interventions for defined patient populations. Evidence-based clinical practice guidelines will ensure that the patients receive high quality care independent of the training of healthcare workers, type of provider, or the health insurance company.

Executive Summary

In this chapter we discussed the status of healthcare and market access of medicines in selected Middle Eastern countries, focusing on the United Arab Emirates (UAE) and highlighting key developments and activities managed by the GCC Executive Office and implemented in the GCC, Jordan, Lebanon, and Egypt. A general outlook of the healthcare system and health policies in these countries is presented. In addition, discussion of the pathways of market access of new medicines including regulation, pricing and reimbursement processes (where applicable) are summarized.

Market access to new medicines can hold both challenges and catalyzers. Challenges include barriers to the use of economic evaluation in policy decision-making in Middle Eastern countries that can be overcome by: standardizing economic evaluation methods, publishing economic evaluations, educating stakeholders including decision-makers, health professionals, and the public, making the economic evaluation processes transparent and participatory, and incorporating other health preferences into the decision-making framework such as equity, necessity, and social solidarity.

The catalyzers of market access are focused on the UAE. For instance, Public-Private Partnerships will continue to play an important role in driving growth in the UAE's and ME healthcare sectors. Top priorities in the UAE's government agenda include quality education, healthcare reform, mandatory healthcare insurance coverage for the whole population, and rational market access pathways of medical technologies based on cost-effectiveness criteria without delaying registration and access by patients, and enhancing the UAE's competitiveness through increased investments in research and biotechnology.

Examples of successful market access strategies are presented and future adaptations of these strategies are highlighted.

The future expansion of access to medicines in the Middle-East and in particular the UAE will depend on:

- public private partnerships;
- availability of data;
- implementation of pharmacoeconomic guidelines; and
- integration of best available evidence in clinical practice.

6.10 Acknowledgements

The efforts and feedback offered in the development of this chapter by the ISPOR UAE Chapter members is much appreciated.

ISPOR UAE Chapter members represent different stakeholders, such as academia, regulator, health provider, industry, and health insurance companies.

The following individuals are recognized for providing input and offering assistance and constructive feedback throughout the process that led to shaping the final document: Dr. Antoine El Khoury, Dr. Naam Jamshed, Dr. Kasem Akhras, Dr. Fady Robehmed, Dr. Sebastian Garrido, Dr. Mohammed Tannira, Dr. Ihab Shahin, Dr. John Gamil Mikhail, Dr. Shadi Elias, and Dr. Hany Hanser.

The following individuals are recognized for reviewing, proofing and providing input: Dr. Osama Hussein Mohammed, Dr. João Carapinha, and Dr. Amad Al Azzawi.

A special thanks goes to Dr. Mubarak Al Ameri for his valuable input and active support in this project and to Dr. Lara Qatami, who has been instrumental in collecting data, and conducting participant interviews of key industry figures as a way to validate data, and to Dr. Sanah Hasan for her countless efforts in reviewing, proofing, editing multiple drafts of this chapter and for giving valuable feedback into the completion of this project.

6.11 References

1. Middle East. Available at https://en.wikipedia.org/wiki/Middle_East (last accessed December 2015)
2. The World Bank. Countries and Economies. http://data.worldbank.org/country (last accessed December 2015)
3. The Cooperation Council for the Arab States of the Gulf. Available at http://www.gcc-sg.org/eng/ (last accessed December 2015)
4. The Executive Board of the Health Ministers' Council for GCC States. Available at http://sgh.org.sa/en-us/home.aspx (last accessed December 2015)
5. World Health Organization. United Arab Emirates. Health Profile 2013. Available at http://www.who.int/countries/are/en/ (last accessed December 2015)

6. United Arab Emirates. National Bureau of Statistics. Available at www.uaestatistics. gov.ae (last accessed December 2015)

7. Al Ahdab OG. Pros & Cons of Pricing and Reimbursement Systems in Saudi Arabia, Egypt, United Arab Emirates, Qatar and Jordan. UAE Profile, ISPOR Arabic Network Forum, 2-6 Jun 2012, DC, USA. Available at http://www.ispor. org/meetings/WashingtonDC0512/releasedpresentations/ISPOR-DC-2012-Ola-Ghaleb-DC-4-June-2012.pdf (last accessed December 2015)

8. UAE National Bureau of Statistics. Open Data for United Arab Emirates. Available at http://opendata.nbs.gov.ae/?lang=en (last accessed December 2015)

9. World Health Organization. United Arab Emirates. Country Cooperation Strategy at a glance. 2014. Available at http://www.who.int/countryfocus/cooperation_ strategy/ccsbrief_are_en.pdf (last accessed December 2015)

10. Business Monitoring International (BMI) Report 2014

11. Business Monitoring International (BMI) Report 2009

12. US-UAE Business Council. The UAE Healthcare Sector. Available at http://usuaebusiness.org/wp-content/uploads/2014/06/HealthcareReport_ Update_June2014.pdf (last accessed December 2015)

13. UAE Government Vision 2021. Available at http://www.vision2021.ae/en (last accessed December 2015)

14. UAE Competitiveness Council. Available at http://www.ecc.ae/competitiveness/ uae-current-standing (last accessed December 2015)

15. United Arab Emirates. Ministry of Health. Available at http://www.moh.gov.ae/en/ pages/default.aspx?sw=1 (last accessed December 2015)

16. Health Authority - Abu Dhabi. Available at http://www.haad.ae/Haad/ (last accessed December 2015)

17. Dubai Health Authority. Available at https://www.dha.gov.ae/en/pages/dhahome. aspx (last accessed December 2015)

18. Sharjah Healthcare City. Available at http://www.shcc.gov.ae/ (last accessed December 2015)

19. United Arab Emirates. Ministry of Finance. Available at www.mof.gov.ae (last accessed December 2015)

20. Abu Dhabi Health Services SEHA. Available at https://www.seha.ae/English/pages/ default.aspx (last accessed December 2015)

21. Cleveland Clinic Abu Dhabi. Available at https://www.clevelandclinicabudhabi.ae/ en/pages/default.aspx (last accessed December 2015)

22. Daman Health. Available at https://www.damanhealth.ae/opencms/opencms/ Daman/en/home/ (last accessed December 2015)

23. Pharmaceutical Industry touching new horizons. Oman Economic Review, 2002

24. The World Bank. GDP per capita. Available at http://data.worldbank.org/indicator/ NY.GDP.PCAP.CD/countries?display=default (last accessed December 2015)

25. International Monetary fund, World economic Outlook database, October 2007. https://www.imf.org/external/pubs/ft/weo/2007/02/weodata/index.aspx (last accessed December 2015)

26. World Health Organization. Health Accounts. Country information. Available at http://www.who.int/nha/country/en/2007 (last accessed December 2015)
27. Kasteng F, Wilking N, Jönsson B. Patient Access to Cancer Drugs in Nine Countries in the Middle East. Available at http://www.comparatorreports.se/Middle%20East%20oncology%20drug%20uptake%20Final%20report%20Sept%2015%20 2008.pdf (last accessed December 2015)
28. Frost & Sullivan and Insights Middle East. Report, 2014
29. Al-Saggabi AH. Pros & Cons of Pricing and Reimbursement: Saudi Arabia, Health Care System. ISPOR Arabic Network Forum, 2-6 Jun 2012, DC, USA. Available at http://www.ispor.org/meetings/WashingtonDC0512/releasedpresentations/FINAL-Abdulaziz-Al-Saggabi.pdf (last accessed December 2015)
30. World Health Organization. Saudi Arabia. Health Profile. Available at http://www.who.int/countries/sau/en/ (last accessed December 2015)
31. Alabbadi I. Pros & Cons of Pricing and Reimbursement Systems in Saudi Arabia, Egypt, United Arab Emirates, Qatar and Jordan. ISPOR Arabic Network Forum, 2-6 Jun 2012, DC, USA. Available at http://www.ispor.org/meetings/WashingtonDC0512/releasedpresentations/Moderator-Ibrahim--Alabbadi-final.pdf (last accessed December 2015)
32. World Health Organization. Jordan. Health Profile. Available at http://www.who.int/countries/jor/en/ (last accessed December 2015)
33. Business Monitor International (BMI) Report Q3 2015, Jordan Pharmaceuticals & Healthcare
34. Jordan Food & Drug Administration (JFDA). Available at https://www.healthresearchweb.org/en/jordan/institution_379 (last accessed December 2015)
35. World Health Organization. Egypt. Health Profile. Available at http://www.who.int/countries/egy/en/ (last accessed December 2015)
36. International Society for Pharmacoeconomics and Outcomes Research. ISPOR Global Health Care Systems Road Map. Available at https://www.ispor.org/HTARoadMaps/EgyptPH.asp (last accessed December 2015)
37. World Health Organization. Lebanon. Health Profile. Available at http://www.who.int/countries/lbn/en/ (last accessed December 2015)
38. Ministry of Public Health. Lebanon. Available at http://www.moph.gov.lb/Drugs/Pages/Drugs.aspx (last accessed December 2015)
39. Meyer-Reumann & Partners. Lex Arabiae. Healthcare in Lebanon. Available at http://lexarabiae.meyer-reumann.com/blog/2010-2/healthcare-in-lebanon/ (last accessed December 2015)
40. Business Monitoring International (BMI) Report Q2-2015. Lebanon Pharmaceuticals & Healthcare
41. Edwards LD, Fox AW, Stonier PD. Drug Registration and Pricing in the Middle East. In: Principles and Practice of Pharmaceutical Medicine, 2nd Edition. New York (NY): John Wiley & Sons, 2007
42. Market access for cancer drugs and the role of health economics. Ann Oncol 2007: 18 (suppl 3); iii55-66

43. Sullivan SD, Kanavos P, Kaló Z. Principle of External Price Referencing . Under submission
44. Middle East & Africa Pharma & Healthcare Insight Business Monitor International, 2007
45. Kaló Z, Alabbadi I, Al Ahdab OG, Al-Badriyeh D, et al. Implications of external price referencing of pharmaceuticals in Middle East countries. *Expert Rev Pharmacoecon Outcomes Res* 2015; 15: 993-8
46. MOH UAE Continuous Professional Development Pharma. Available at www.cpd-pharma.ae (last accessed December 2015)
47. Business Monitor International (BMI). Pharmaceuticals and Healthcare Industry Forecasts. 2007-2008.
48. Al Ahdab O, Younes N, Albraiki, F, et al. CIF price comparative study. Ministry of Health, UAE, 2010
49. MOH UAE Continuous Professional Development Pharma. Innovative Medicines Price Reduction, 2015
50. WAM Emirates News Agency. Ministry of Health launches 5th initiative to reduce prices of 422 innovative drug items. 2014. Available at http://www.wam.ae/en/news/economics/1395270177191.html (last accessed December 2015)
51. Drug Department Data Records. Ministry of Health, UAE, 2015
52. Ghaleb Al Ahdab O. Managed Entry Agreements (Mea) In Egypt, Lebanon, Saudi Arabia, And United Arab Emirates. Arabica Network Forum, 2015. Available at www.ispor.org/Event/GetReleasedPresentation/325 (last accessed December 2015)
53. Central Gulf Committee for Drug Registration. Registration By-Laws of Pharmaceutical Companies and Their Products. Available at http://www.sgh.org.sa/Portals/0/PDF/Cen_registration/Registration%20By-Laws%20of%20Pharmaceutical%20Companies%20and%20Their%20Products.pdf (last accessed December 2015)
54. Saudi Food & Drug Authority. Available at http://www.sfda.gov.sa/en/Pages/default.aspx (last accessed December 2015)
55. Hajed M. Hajed. Saudi Pricing Guidelines and The Proposed New Pricing System. Saudi Food and Drug Authority (SFDA). Available at http://www.sfda.gov.sa/ar/news/Documents/SaudiPricingGuidelinesandTheProposedNewSystem.pdf (last accessed December 2015)
56. National Organization for Drug Control And Research (NODCAR). Available at http://www.nodcar.eg.net/main/ (last accessed December 2015)
57. Clancy CM, Eisenberg JM. Outcomes Research: Measuring the End Results of Health Care. *Science* 1998; 282: 245-46
58. Drummond MF, Sculpher MJ, Torrance G, et al. Methods for the Economic Evaluation of Health Care Programmes. (3rd ed.) New York: Oxford University Press, 2005: 1
59. Szabo SM, Osenenko KM, Qatami L, et al. Quality of care for type 2 Diabetes Mellitus in Duba: Hedis-like assessment. *Int J Endocrinol* 2015; 2015: 413276

60. Yothasamut J, Tantivess S, Teerawattananon Y. Using Economic Evaluation in Policy Decision-Making in Asian Countries: Mission Impossible or Mission Probable? *Value Health*.2009; 12 Suppl 3: S26-30

61. Shafrin J. Cost of drug development: $1 billion. Healthcare Economist, 2010. Available at http://healthcare-economist.com/2010/02/16/cost-of-drug-development-1-billion/ (last accessed December 2015)

62. The use of external reference pricing, Pharmaceutical pricing, 2013, RAND Europe

63. Axios International. Available at http://axios-group.com/axiosinternational/work (last accessed December 2015)

64. Ringborg A, Cropet C, Jonsson B, et al. Resource use associated with type 2 diabetes in Asia, Latin America, the Middle East and Africa: results from the International Diabetes Management Practices Study (IDMPS). *Int J Clin Pract* 2009; 63: 997-1007

65. International Diabetes Federation. Atlas 2014. Available at http://www.idf.org

66. UAE National Diabetes Committee, National clinical Guidelines, 2009

67. Dubai Standards in Healthcare 2015

68. Dubai Health Authority launches Dubai Standards of Healthcare for diabetes management. Wam – Emirates News Agency, 2015. Available at https://www.wam.ae/en/news/emirates/1395277998948.html (last accessed December 2015)

69. Dubai adopts standardised diabetes care protocol. Gulf News Health, 2015. Available at http://gulfnews.com/news/uae/health/dubai-adopts-standardised-diabetes-care-protocol-1.1472480 (last accessed December 2015)

70. Dubai Health Authority's new standards to tackle diabetes. The National, 2015. Available at http://www.thenational.ae/uae/health/dubai-health-authoritys-new-standards-to-tackle-diabetes (last accessed December 2015)

71. Asma Ali Zain. Managed Entry Agreements (Mea) In Egypt, Lebanon, Saudi Arabia, And United Arab Emirates. Khaleej Times, 2015. Available at http://www.khaleejtimes.com/nation/uae-health/basic-insurance-in-dubai-to-cover-diabetes (last accessed December 2015)

72. Egypt opens first factory for locally produced Sovaldi. HCV New Drug Research. Available at http://hepatitiscnewdrugs.blogspot.ae/2015/05/egypt-opens-first-factory-for-locally.html (last accessed December 2015)

73. AMCP Concept Series Paper on Disease Management. Available at http://www.amcp.org/WorkArea/DownloadAsset.aspx?id=9295 (last accessed December 2015)

7. Market Access in Sub-Saharan Africa countries

Debra Leong, Mark Banfield, Anne Smart

.1 Regional Considerations for Sub-Saharan African Countries and South Africa as a Case Study

The African region has over 892 million inhabitants in 47 countries, accounting for about 12% of the world's population. Africa's pharmaceutical industry increased from approximately US$ 4.7 billion in 2003 to US$ 20.8 billion (retail price) in 2013, and by 2016 pharmaceutical spending on the continent is expected to reach US$ 30 billion, growing at a 10.6% growth rate [1,2]. Although the market potential is significant, the African region presents a multifaceted collection of markets with vast diversity and complex unity. This juxtaposition is underscored by the array of trading blocs known as the Regional Economic Communities (RECs), which bring together individual countries in sub-regions to pursue greater economic integration. There are eight RECs that are considered to be the building blocks of the African economic community, in Figure 1 are shown the main one (Figure 1).

Each REC has similar goals of fostering cooperation and a degree of economic integration, but a number of overlapping countries between the RECs, and politically complicated environments, add significant complexity to this mandate. Despite that, the RECs present an opportunity for harmonization of certain market access pathways. The East African Community (EAC), the most mature REC with the highest sales growth, is progressing on a harmonized approach to medicine evaluation and registration. This suggests that although significant variations may exist with regard to the maturity of national health policies and plans, health financing systems and the pathways to market access, pockets of opportunity still exist.

Sub-Saharan Africa is the region of Africa, south of the Sahara desert in North Africa. The region differentiates itself from North Africa, which is considered a part of the Arab world. Within sub-Saharan Africa, the major markets are South Africa, Nigeria, Kenya and Botswana (in order of pharmaceutical market size). Each is characterized by having a unique healthcare financing system (Table 1) that presents different opportunities and challenges.

The main challenge to harmonization across the region is the different stages in development and implementation in each sub-region and National Medicines Regulatory Authorities. Reference is made to the World Health Organization Prequalification Process which is important in expediting market access for high priority medicines in Africa [5].

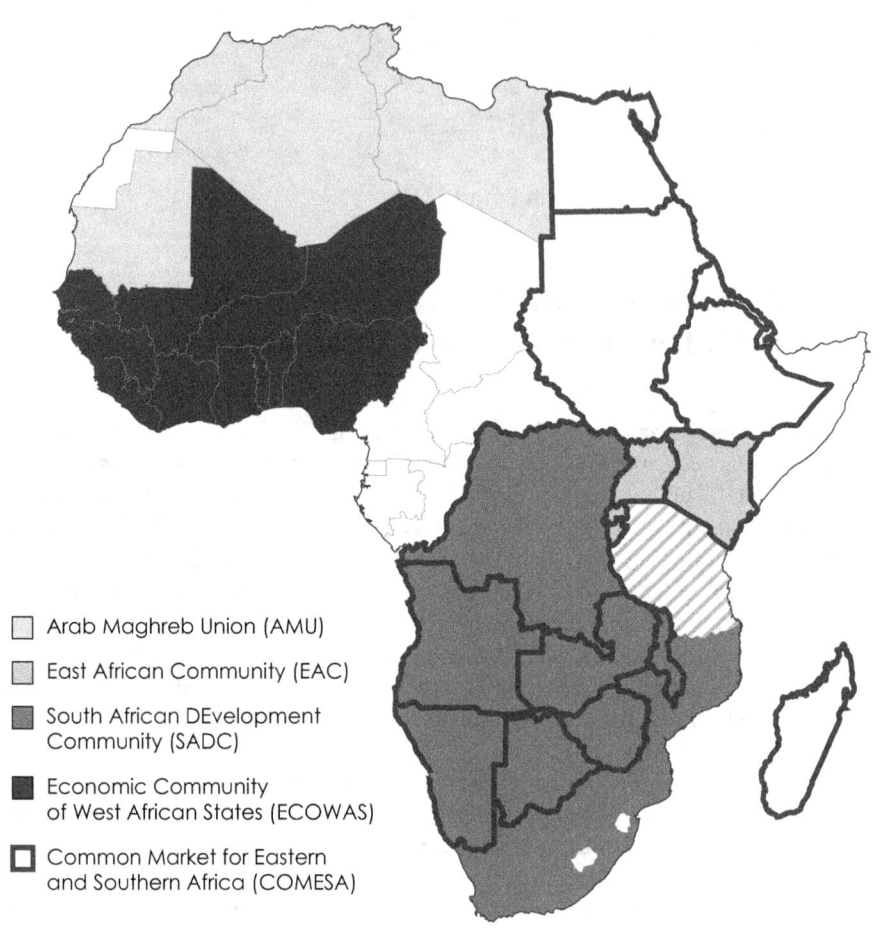

Arab Maghreb Union (AMU)

East African Community (EAC)

South African DEvelopment Community (SADC)

Economic Community of West African States (ECOWAS)

Common Market for Eastern and Southern Africa (COMESA)

Figure 1. Example Regional Economic Communities (RECs) in Africa [3]

Country	Total Healthcare Expenditure (% of GDP)	Public Health Expenditure (% of THE)	Out-of-Pocket Health Expenditure (% of Private Expenditure on Health)	Pharmaceutical Market Size (US$ million)
South Africa	8.9	48.4	13.8	3,700
Nigeria	3.9	27.6	95.8	1,800
Kenya	4.5	41.7	76.6	659
Botswana	5.4	57.1	12.7	56

Table 1. Sub-Saharan Africa Country Health Statistics [2,4]
GDP = Gross Domestic Product; THE = Total Healthcare Expenditure

South Africa represents the biggest pharmaceutical market in sub-Saharan Africa, as well as all of Africa, and growth in this country has been driven by an increasing investment in health system infrastructure to increase access. Total Healthcare Expenditure (THE) in South Africa is 8.9% of Gross Domestic Product (GDP), representing approximately US$ 31 billion in 2013. In the West, Nigeria has the largest population in Africa accompanied by an above average GDP growth rate since 2006. Furthermore, the Nigerian government launched the National Health Insurance Scheme in 2008 with the goal of universal health coverage, although coverage is still low and the urban slums remain underserved. In the East, Kenya has committed to spending 15% of its national budget on healthcare as part of its plan to transition to a middle income country by 2030. As part of the EAC, Kenya also represents a potential opportunity for lower regulatory hurdles to entry. Lastly, Botswana is a small, but relatively wealthy country with a strong national commitment to healthcare. The government report spending more than 15% of its budget on healthcare and public funds currently represent 80% of total health expenditure [6].

While many emerging markets face the increasing burden of chronic Non-Communicable Diseases (NCDs), such as diabetes, cardiovascular disease, and cancer, due to lifestyle and diet trends, the African region faces the particular problem of an increasing burden of NCDs in combination with continuing high morbidity and mortality from communicable diseases. As such, African health systems are faced with significant and evolving challenges to not only address the growing prevalence of NCDs, but also the existing concerns of communicable diseases, and all of this in the context of limited and often inequitably distributed resources. The 2006 World Health Report stated that Africa has 24% of the world's burden of disease, but only 3% of the world's health workers, commanding less than 1% of the world's health expenditure. As a result, Africa has lagged behind the rest of the world on indicators of health, even when compared to other lower income emerging markets. Africans live an average of 14 years less than the average world

	Life Expectancy at Birth, Years (2011)	Adult Mortality Rate per 1000 Population (2011)	Under-5 Mortality Rate per 1000 Live Births (2012)	Maternal Mortality Ratio per 100,000 Live Births (2010)
Africa	56	339	95	480
Southeast Asia	67	194	50	200
Eastern Mediterranean	68	154	57	210
Western Pacific	76	132	16	49
Americas	76	125	15	63
Europe	76	101	12	20
Global	70	160	48	210

Table 2. Health Indicators by WHO Region [1]

citizen. The maternal mortality rate and the mortality rate for children younger than five years are more than double the world average (Table 2).

Furthermore, progress on health indicators is slower than in any other region, suggesting that Africa will continue to lag behind the rest of the world on health indicators for many years to come.

One of the most important reasons for the poor health outcomes in Africa is the way in which healthcare is funded. Even high income countries struggle with rising healthcare costs and this problem is even more acute in Africa due to the scarcity of funds. In 2010, the average Total Health Expenditure per capita was US$ 135 in Africa compared to US$ 3,150 in high income countries. Healthcare funding in Africa is characterized by inconsistent and low public spending, heavy reliance on foreign donors, and significant dependence on out-of-pocket patient payments. African government budgets are often insufficient to address the significant healthcare demands and are further impacted by corruption. Aid coming from external sources is usually inefficiently targeted, focusing disproportionately on high profile conditions, such as HIV/AIDs and malaria, while neglecting other important public health issues, such as infant and maternal mortality that impact a larger proportion of the population. Additionally, the significant reliance on out-of-pocket spending by patients places the greatest burden on the poorest individuals in Africa. In about half of African countries, out-of-pocket (OOP) payments comprises over 40% of THE.

Corruption is a compounding factor in this equation for African countries. The Corruption Perceptions Index scores countries worldwide on how corrupt their public sectors are perceived to be on a scale of 0 (highly corrupt) to 100 (very clean). The index is currently lower than 50 in 91% of African countries [7-9]. The root of this corruption is lack of accountability and absence of controls on medical substances. Once foreign aid funding goes through the public health ministries, there is little or no system to keep track of how the money flows or where it is allocated. Corruption plays a major role in African healthcare systems at the government, hospital and even healthcare provider level. The impact of corruption on the healthcare system is low returns on health investments and impedance to the access and quality of patient care.

7.2 Kenya

Kenya is representative of the East African Community approach towards medicines and medical device regulation and harmonization. The Kenya Pharmacy and Poisons Board is responsible for registering all medical devices, cosmetics, biological products and medicinal products, conforming to the Essential Principals for safety and performance. Application for registration of Medicinal products is initiated by the submission of a Common Technical Dossier (CTD) and registration can take 90 days from application. Medicines are evaluated on a "first in first out" basis and may take 12 months, except for "Priority Medicines" (medicines not available in Kenya for which there is a public health need) which may be fast tracked.

In Kenya, the pathways to market access to both the public and private sectors are unstructured. Access to the public sector is based upon procurement and tendering. There are no pricing regulations for medicines or medical devices in Kenya. Since price controls were abolished in 1994, there has been a discussion on the need for re-establishing pricing controls in the healthcare sector to assist in achieving Kenya's Vision 2030 Development Goals. Procurement in the public sector is regulated by the Public Procurement and Disposal Act, which requires bids to be awarded to the lowest cost product that meets the procuring department's needs. However, the ordinary citizen (*mwananchi*) in Kenya is reliant on the private healthcare system. The Competition Act (2010) regulates the manner in which prices are set in the private sector as 80% of healthcare expenses are private expenditure. It should be noted that products procured on the international market on tender are subject to Verification Of Conformity (VOC) at Import Control, and this should be taken into account when conducting such business.

.3 Nigeria

Nigeria is representative of the ECOWAS (Economic Community Of West African States) region. While a regulatory pathway exists in Nigeria, there is no formal pathway to market access outside of procurement. Medicines and medical devices are regulated by the National Agency for Food and Drug Administration and Control (NAFDAC), under the federal government of Nigeria. Healthcare products are registered on the Nigerian Automated Product and Monitoring Solutions (NAPAMS) system online, with support of a CTD. Registration takes 100 workdays after submission of samples for evaluation. There are no legal or regulatory provisions affecting pricing of medicines, medical devices, and associated healthcare products.

.4 South Africa

This chapter examines South Africa as a more detailed case study for Sub-Saharan Africa and also as the largest market in Africa.

South Africa has a population of 52.8 million inhabitants and a GDP of US$ 683 million (both 2013), making it the 6th most populous country and highest GDP in the African region [1]. The country has been a constitutional democracy since 1994 and is divided into nine provinces, each with a Provincial Legislature and their own Department Of Health (DOH). While South Africa is considered a "middle income" developing country, the country has faced challenges with regard to human and social capital development, which are indicated by the high unemployment rate, persistent high levels of poverty, and the increasing income inequality between the rich and the poor. WorldBank 2011 statistics suggested that 53.8% of the total South African population still resides below the national poverty line, with this proportion increasing to more than 75% for the rural population. Furthermore, the Gini index, which is a measure of income distribution, was 0.65 in 2011 in South Africa, among the highest (and most inequitable) in the world [10]. Altogether, these statistics suggest that understanding market access in South Africa requires the consideration of a vastly varied population with a very different willingness and ability to spend on healthcare.

According to 2013 statistics from the WHO, life expectancy in South Africa has increased from 54 years in 2005 to 60 years in 2011 and infant mortality has decreased from 58 per 1000 live births in 2002 to 34 per 1000 live births in 2014 [11]. These overall health outcome improvements are partly due to the introduction of new innovations, rapid expansion of treatments for HIV/AIDs and tuberculosis (TB), and expanded access to immunization. However, communicable diseases, such as TB, HIV, and malaria, still remain prevalent and contribute about 50% of significant morbidity and mortality. South Africa still has one of the highest TB incidence rates in the world (1 per 100 population), with two of three TB patients also contracting HIV. In addition, HIV/AIDS remains the leading cause of death, responsible for over 200,000 deaths in 2012. Furthermore, greater overall spending power and the expanding middle class in South Africa have led to

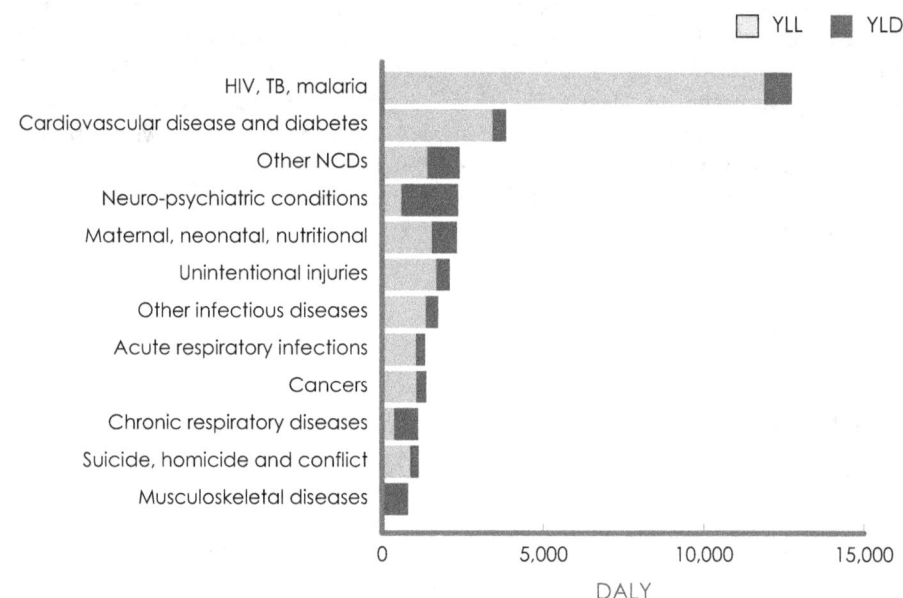

Figure 2. Burden of Disease in South Africa, 2012. Disability-Adjusted Life Years (DALYs) are the sum of Years of Life Lost to premature mortality (YLL) and Years of healthy life Lost due to Disability (YLD) [12]
NCD = Non-Communicable Disease; TB = Tuberculosis

changes in lifestyle and diet that contribute to the growing prevalence of NCDs. For example, increased alcohol consumption, increased consumption of packaged foods, and decreased physical activity are all risk factors contributing to NCDs. In fact, the probability of premature mortality from NCDs between the ages of 30 and 70 years is now 43% in South Africa, compared to 48% due to communicable, maternal, perinatal and nutritional conditions [11]. Burden of disease in South Africa is represented in Figure 2.

General Outlook of Healthcare System and Health Policies

The National Health Act 2003 [13] provides a framework for a single health system in South Africa. It highlights the rights and responsibilities of healthcare providers and users, and ensures broader community participation in healthcare delivery, from local health facilities up to the national level. It establishes provincial health services and outlines the general functions of provincial health departments. South Africa spends approximately 8.9% of GDP on healthcare [4]. While this is more than most middle income developing countries, health outcomes remain poor when compared to similar developing countries and this has been attributed to the inequities between the public and private sectors. Although public health spending has increased at an annual rate of 7.6% since 2001, the majority of funding has gone to non-hospital care.

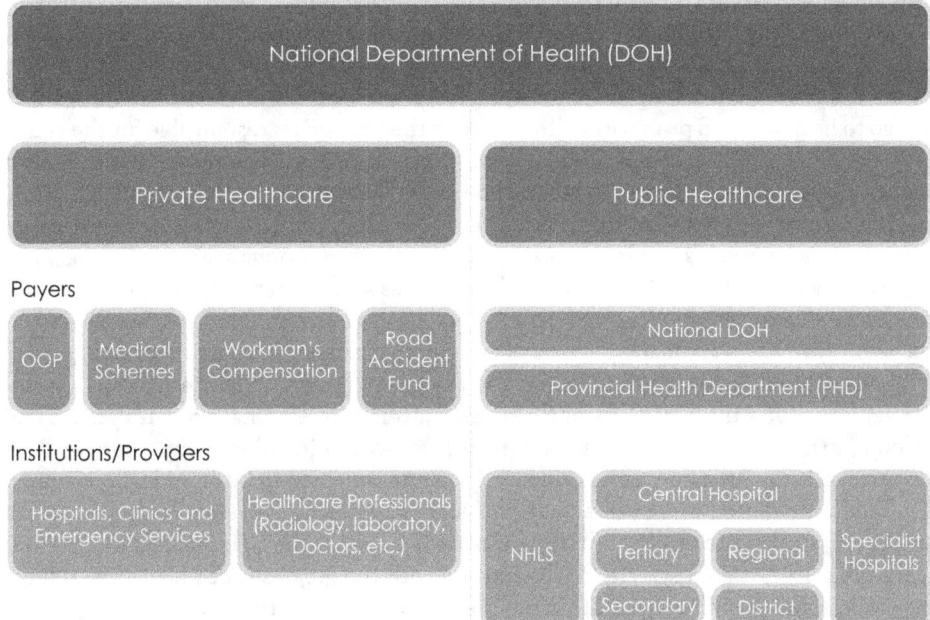

Figure 3. Structure of South Africa Health System
NHLS = National Health Laboratory Service; OOP = Out-Of-Pocket

The overall structure of the healthcare system in South Africa is outlined in Figure 3.

The national Department of Health is responsible for all healthcare in South Africa. The South African healthcare financing system is characterized by a dichotomy that exists between the public and private sectors, with inequitable distribution of resources relative to covered populations and disease burden. The public sector serves an estimated 84% of the population and comprises approximately 49% of THE, while the private sector serves the wealthier 16% of the population who can afford it, but makes up more than half (51%) of THE [14]. As a result, there are profound inequalities that exist in the quality of services provided by public and private healthcare. The private sector has resources similar to those available in Western Europe, while the public sector has resources comparable to countries of much lower economic status. Most public health facilities are directly owned and managed by the Provincial Health Departments (PHDs), while most private health facilities are for-profit commercial organizations. The private sector is highly concentrated and is dominated by three hospital groups (NetCare, Mediclinic, Life Group), accounting for 87% of private beds [15].

Most health services in the public sector are still being funded by the government, although a National Health Insurance (NHI) program is being implemented in an effort to improve the quality and equity of healthcare provision. Currently, however, public healthcare is funded through progressive general taxation and the national government sets the overall healthcare budget and establishes allocations for provinces. Allocations are then distributed according to province population, but take into account the percentage of the provincial population not covered by private medical schemes (Gauteng and KwaZulu-Natal are the highest funded provinces). Provinces are responsible for deciding on the amount of their annual budget that will be allocated to healthcare and what share of that will go to hospitals and primary healthcare, with the nine PHDs responsible for the actual provision of care. Government funded services include primary healthcare, basic curative services, and specialist services in central hospitals. Patients pay a user fee, which is set by the DOH according to the Uniform Patient Fee Schedule (UPFS) and on a sliding scale according to each patient's income. However, substantial exemptions are made for the poorer patients who predominantly use the public services sector since there is no incentive for fee collection as revenue is remitted. As a result, physicians often charge patients based on their ability to pay, with many physicians receiving no payment for their services.

The latest and most significant reform to the health system in South Africa is the implementation of a the NHI system, which is an attempt to eliminate the disparities and inequities that exist between the public and private sectors in order to improve overall access to quality healthcare services. The NHI scheme launched in 2011 and will be implemented over a period of 14 years, with the goal of providing universal health insurance and quality healthcare to all South African citizens by 2025. The NHI system aims to eliminate the current tiered system in which those with the greatest need have the least access to care and poorer health outcomes. The NHI will address this through:

- improved cross-subsidization in the overall health system, whereby funding contributions are linked to an individual's ability to pay and benefits are in line with an individual's need for care; and

- free provision of broad benefits to all citizens at the point of service with free choice of provider within a district.

In addition, the NHI system will also call for the eventual transition of the current antiquated global budget hospital payment scheme towards a case-based payment system using DRGs (Diagnosis Related Groups). The NHI will function as the sole payer and is funded through general tax revenue and progressive employee/employer contributions over a set income level. Covered healthcare services will be provided through contracted public and private providers. To date, NHI has been piloted in 11 districts and currently covers 11 million individuals or about 21% of the South African population [16].

In contrast to public sector funding, private health insurance in South Africa accounts for approximately half of THE, but access to the private sector has been limited to the wealthier upper class due to escalating premium levels. Medical schemes, administrators, and managed care organizations are regulated by the Council for Medical Schemes (CMS) that legislates maximum annual member fee increases, Prescribed Minimum Benefits (PMB), and minimum reserve funds. The medical schemes or funds operate on a not-for-profit basis, but contract for-profit organizations to administer the care on behalf of members. Financing of private insurance plans differs, but commonly consists of annual fees, a set deductible, and various co-pays. Membership is disproportionately concentrated in Gauteng, KwaZulu-Natal, and Western Cape, which together account for over 65% of covered lives. Annual premiums paid by the patient in the private sector average US$ 172 per member and premium levels have increased at a rate of approximately 13.7% per year, resulting in private health insurance being mostly limited to the upper class. While gap funding and hospital insurance have emerged in the private sector in recent years, they still only play a small role [17].

In South Africa, 87 private medical schemes currently exist with around 8.7 million beneficiaries, accounting for approximately 16% of the population. Only 30 schemes are estimated to have over 30,000 beneficiaries, with Discovery Health being the largest scheme and functioning largely as a gatekeeper to the private sector. These schemes have a total annual contribution flow of about R 129.8 billion or US$ 9.4 billion. However, the number of medicals schemes has been decreasing over the past decade, from over 120 schemes in 2004 to the current number of 87 at the end of 2013. This is likely due to significant consolidation of schemes as a result of the overpricing of private healthcare through the fee-for-service system and the CMS requirements for a minimum annual reserve of 25% of contributions. Smaller medical schemes have been the most adversely impacted, as the number of small schemes (fewer than 6,000 members) has dropped from 37 in 2012 to 32 in 2013 [17].

Despite government funding and private health insurance, approximately 16% of the South Africa population still self-pays for health services in the private sector on an out-of-pocket basis. This mostly consists of primary care from general practitioners, drugs purchased from retail pharmacies and user fees for care in the public sector. It is estimated that OOP payments push about 290,000 households below the poverty line in South Africa in a single year.

Historical inequalities in health spending between the public and private sectors and among different provinces is also reflected in disparities in the quality of the healthcare infrastructure. Currently, the overall level of infrastructure is insufficient to support the healthcare burden in South Africa. 2014 WHO statistics report that 0.08 physicians exist per 1,000 patients in South Africa, which is significantly below the global average of 1.3 physicians per 1,000 patients [1]. The lack of physician resources has continued to worsen with data from the South Africa Health Department showing a 35% year-on-year increase in nurse and doctor job vacancies. A key challenge to this is that South Africa's eight medical schools only produce approximately 200 doctors per year, although a ninth school has been established and is expected to open in 2016. Furthermore, these resource constraints are even more acute in the public sector and rural areas, as around 70% of all physicians and specialists only work in the private sector, which is largely focused in urban areas leaving the rural areas inadequately covered.

Pathways of Market Access (Regulation, Pricing, and Reimbursement)

For a new drug to gain access to the South African market, it must gain regulatory approval, undergo competitive/reference pricing and apply for inclusion to reimbursement lists. Overall, this is a lengthy undertaking, as regulatory approval alone can take as long as three to five years. Separate pricing and reimbursement pathways exist for the public and private sectors with varying stakeholders, requirement and steps for each pathway.

Regulation

The Medicines Control Council (MCC) was founded in 1966 under the Medicines and Related Substances Control Act (Act 101 of 1965) and is responsible for all pharmaceutical products manufactured, imported and marketed in South Africa, including New Chemical Entities (NCEs), multisource (generic) products, product line extensions, and biological medicines. Recent amendments to the Act will cause the MCC to be reconstituted as the South African Health Products Regulatory Authority (SAHPRA), which will be responsible for registering all health products, including pharmaceuticals and devices, in South Africa.

The MCC has a limited in-house staff of approximately 100 people with reliance on various experts from academic institutions. There are approximately 300 registration submissions per year, mostly for generics following patent expiration, with NCE dossiers only comprising 10-15 submissions per year. The limited capacity of the MCC in combination with the significant generic application load has resulted in significant backlogs, with the average time to registration of three to five years [18].

The registration application process is a highly formalized and costly exercise involving the submission of a standardized Common Technical Document (CTD) in person. Comprehensive application guidelines have been published by the MCC to guide this process and applications include labeling data, expert reports, and clinical trial data. Once the MCC receives the CTD, it is evaluated by three expert committees, including the Naming and Scheduling Committee, Pharmaceutical and Analytical and Central Clinical Committees, and the Biological Medicines Committee, before being sent to the MCC council for final approval.

The MCC aligns itself with several foreign regulatory bodies, including the U.S. Food and Drug Administration (FDA), the U.E. European Medicines Agency (EMA and national regulatory authorities), Australian Therapeutic Goods Administration (TGA), the Canadian Health Canada, and the Japanese Ministry of Health, Labor and Welfare (MHLW). Pharmaceutical products that are registered in countries with which the MCC aligns itself can undergo a shortened evaluation timeline known as the Abbreviated Medicine Review Process (AMRP). The AMRP is based mainly on expert reports of the pharmaco-toxicological and clinical data, although it should be noted that the AMRP offers an abbreviated evaluation process, not an abbreviated application.

Under certain circumstances, the MCC may also "fast-track" the registration process for specific medicines that have important therapeutic benefit and which are required urgently to deal with key health problems (e.g., HIV or tuberculosis therapies). Typically, only an NCE that does not appear on the Essential Medicines List (EML) would be considered for the expedited review process. A less comprehensive application is required for this process, including a written notification from the Minister indicating that the medicine is essential to national health, an expert report, and a Summary Basis for Regulatory Action (SBRA). In such cases, the MCC will notify the applicant within 30 days if the application qualifies for the expedited review process and a registration decision can be made within 9 months of application receipt.

Section 21 of the Medicines and Related Substances Control Act allows for products not registered to be used under special conditions for humanitarian purposes. Ad-hoc submissions are made by doctors for use of unregistered items on a named-patient basis. Submissions may include NCEs not yet approved by the MCC but approved by the FDA and EMA, drugs not approved by any regulatory authority, and "unproven" items and medicines previously registered, but later withdrawn by a pharmaceutical company because of a lack of financial viability.

Pricing

South Africa developed a National Drug Policy in 1996, which signaled a multi-faceted series of interventions to reduce medicine prices and also improve prescribing and dispensing practices. Once a drug has gained regulatory approval, the next step is a pricing submission to the National DOH Pricing Committee. Single Exit Price (SEP) is a transparent pricing mechanism in South Africa, which lists the maximum price at which a medicine may be charged. The system was introduced in 2006, and affects all medicines in South Africa with the exception of complimentary medicines, nutraceuticals, vitamins, supplements, and medical devices. Current SEP legislation excludes any discounts, mark-ups, bonuses or free samples in the private sector. This serves to regulate the profits made on the sale of pharmaceuticals to prevent financial incentives for inappropriate use of medicines by physicians. Manufacturers are required to sell their products at a single price, irrespective of volumes. It can take 4-8 weeks to release a SEP and coding for sale in the private sector.

For a new drug, the first SEP is applied for as part of an importer's or manufacturer's initial medicine registration process with the MCC, forming part of the CTD. Applicants have to provide evidence in support of their SEP application as well as other local and international benchmarks. Typically, the lowest country benchmark price will be accepted. Reference pricing is used to limit the price of an individual drug by comparison with the price of other drugs in the same category, based on the same active ingredient, drugs in a pharmacological class, and drugs with a similar therapeutic effect. For new drugs, pharmacoeconomic analyses may be applied to determine SEP, through an evidence-based approach considering both direct and indirect costs. SEPs are supposed to be adjusted annually by way of a notice from the Minister of Health. However, limited adjustments were made in the first few years of SEP and in more recent times SEP has largely followed the base inflation rate, not the medical inflation rate.

Medicine pricing in the public sector is not subject to SEP, but new drugs are expected to be competitively priced to win tenders for medicines. Pricing in the public sector is significantly lower than in the private sector, as tender prices may be up to 90% of the SEP. However, tenders have also increasingly come into use in private sector hospital groups as a mechanism for further price control. In the public sector, the DOH negotiates a tender price with various pharmaceutical companies for drugs used in public hospitals. Drugs on the national tender are on the Essential Medicines List, usually based on the final recommendations of the National Essential Medicines List Committee (NEMLC). Competition between pharmaceutical companies often helps to drive down tender prices substantially and tenders are often given to the most cost-effective in a class of medicines, further increasing competition.

Aside from pricing regulations on drugs, the DOH also enforces fixed fees for wholesalers and pharmacists. Dispensers may charge an additional dispensing fee, depending on the price of the medicine (see Table 3).

Dispensing fees have been revised multiple times in past years due to court challenges from pharmacists who have found these fees unacceptable.

Since the implementation of pricing regulations, overall drug prices have decreased by an average of 19%, with prices for generics reduced by approximately 25% to 30% and prices for originators reduced by approximately 12%. The regulations have also eliminated price discrimination between urban and rural areas and offered greater transparency to consumers, as drug pricing for the SEP is listed on

SEP	Maximum Dispensing Fees*
Less than R 85.69	R 7.04 + 46% SEP
Less than R 228.56	R 18.80 + 33% SEP
Less than R 799.99	R 59.83 + 15% SEP
Greater than or equal to R 799.99	R 150 + 5% SEP

Table 3. Maximum dispensing fees based on Single Exit Price (SEP) [19]
*Exclusive of 14% VAT

the South African Medicine Price Registry (MPR) website. However, these stringent pricing regulations have faced significant opposition from manufacturers, medical practitioners, wholesalers, and pharmacists. In particular, the most significant challenge has been determining a reasonable and enforceable dispensing fee for pharmacists and this remains highly contested.

Reimbursement – Public Sector

The Essential Medicines Programme (EMP) of South Africa was implemented in 1996 with the aim of providing equal access to medicines for all South Africans. The key components of the EMP are the Essential Medicines List and the Standard Treatment Guidelines (STGs). The EML is based on the WHO guidelines for essential medicines, which are those that "satisfy the priority healthcare needs of the population" and are "intended to be available within the context of functioning health systems at all times in adequate quantities, in the appropriate dosage forms, with assured quality and adequate information, and at a price the individual and community can afford" [20]. The EML provides a national formulary for three levels of care: primary, secondary, and hospital-level. It forms the cornerstone of drug funding for the public sector in South Africa. In 2012, the first online edition of the Tertiary and Quarternary Care EML was published for use at tertiary provincial or quaternary (academic) hospitals.

Although South Africa's EML is based off the WHO's EML, some interesting distinctions exist when comparing the two lists. The number of medicines for NCDs is higher in the South African EML than the WHO EML (91 in South Africa vs. 63 in WHO), suggesting that there is a recognition and effort to address the growing burden of NCDs within the country. However, the number of oncology drugs is significantly less than the number in the WHO EML (4 in South Africa vs. 30 in WHO). This is consistent with a lower prioritization of cancer in national health priorities compared to communicable diseases and other NCDs, such as diabetes [21].

The ministerial-appointed National Essential Medicines List Committee is responsible for developing and revising the EML, under the advisement of its Expert Review Committees. These review committees are comprised of a mix of experts with clinical, process, and methodological knowledge. The process for EML inclusion is outlined in Figure 4.

To apply for addition to the EML, the sponsor first submits a dossier to the National DOH. The NEMLC reviews drugs for the availability of robust, high quality evidence regarding efficacy, effectiveness, and safety. A pharmacoeconomic analysis is not formally required for evaluation, although some success has been achieved with the application of such analyses. One example is the pharmacoeconomic analysis of capecitabine for the treatment of metastatic colorectal cancer, which led to funding approval in 2012. Following approval of addition to the EML, the sponsor submits a pricing tender to the Tender Committee within the DOH. If a tender is not approved, the sponsor can resubmit the tender with a lower price. After tender approval, the NEMLC makes a final funding decision. The NEMLC review process can take 60-120 business days and the tendering process can take approximately 100 business days, resulting in a total of 160-220 business days, or 8-11 months, for a funding decision to be made.

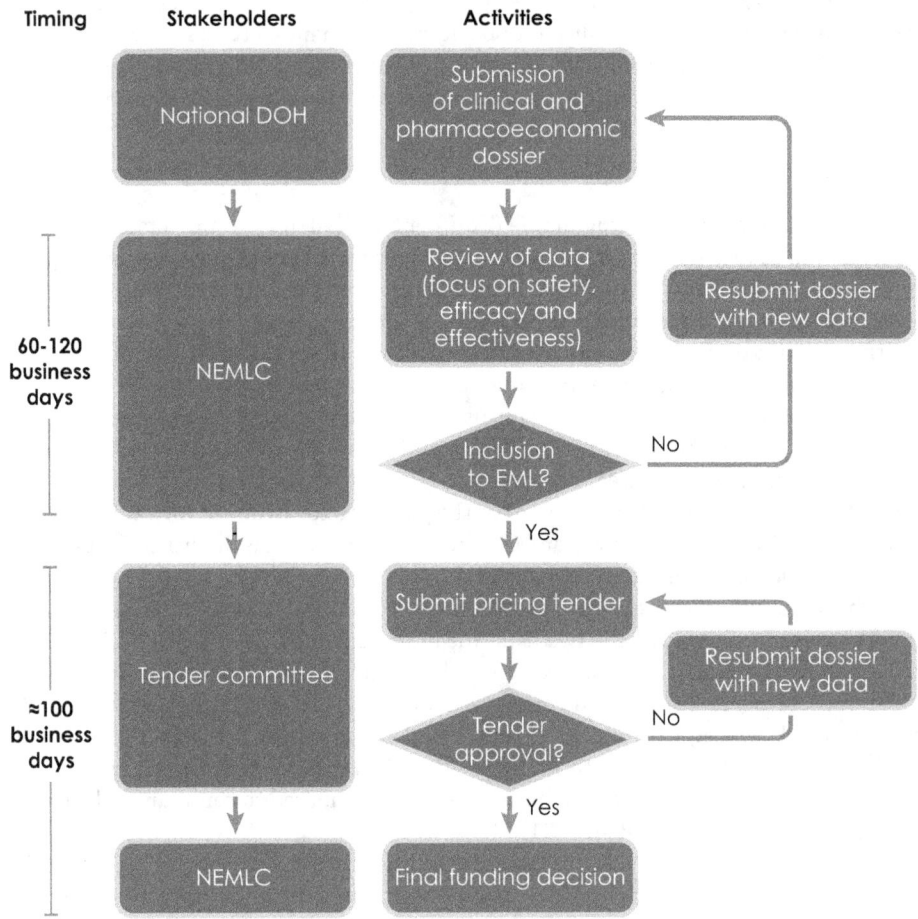

Figure 4. Essential Medicines List (EML) Approval Process [22]
DOH = Department of Health; EML = Essential Medicines List; NEMLC = National Essential Medicines List Committee

The Pharmacy and Therapeutics Committees (PTCs) are provincial-, district- and facility-based committees that have the mandate of ensuring rational, efficient, and cost-effective supply and use of medicines. The PTCs are responsible for supporting the implementation of the EML and STGs by developing a formulary list that provides prescribers and dispensers with information on the medicines authorized for use within their jurisdiction. The provincial Pharmacy and Therapeutics Committees have a degree of autonomy with regard to medicine selection and are able to make selections of medicines not included on the EML that are funded from provincial budgets. However, there is no formal central advisory body to apply evidence-based and health economic principles to the rec-

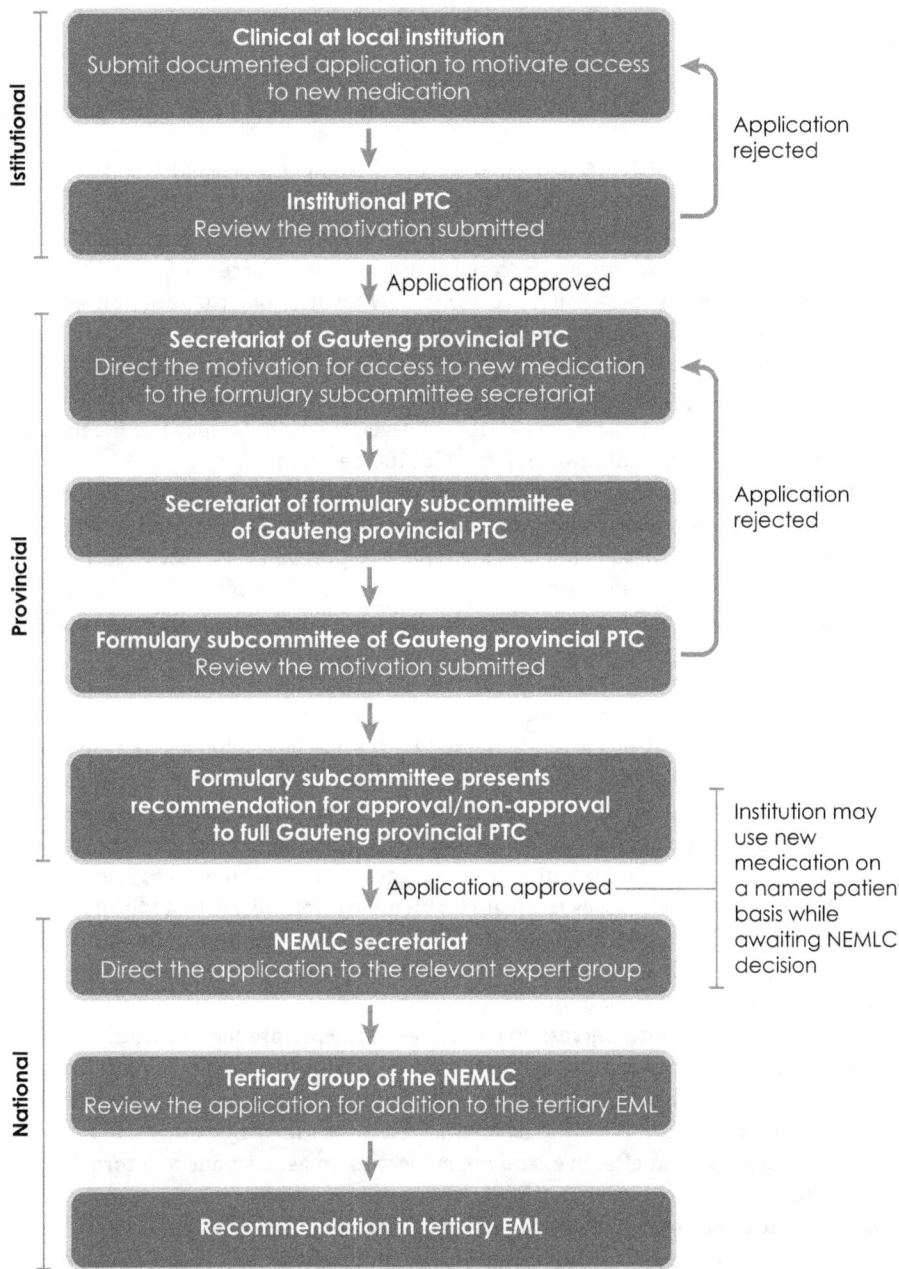

Figure 5. Gauteng PTC Formulary Application Process for Non-EML Medicine [23]
EML = Essential Medicines List; NEMLC = National Essential Medicines List Committee;
PTC = Pharmacy and Therapeutics Committee

ommendation, resulting in a variable selection process and outcome from province to province, resulting in inequitable access. This is amplified by the fact that PTC development progress has been patchy throughout the country, with Gauteng, Western Cape, and KwaZulu-Natal identified as being more successful than other provinces in medicine selection.

The provincial PTC is also influenced by district and hospital-based PTCs. For a medicine that is not on the EML or provincial formulary, an addition to the formulary may be driven by a clinician with the necessary supporting evidence. As an example, the Gauteng Provincial PTC has a standardized process for application to access of non-EML items whereby local institutions can request access to new medications that are non-EML and non-Gauteng Medicine Formulary items (Figure 5).

The application for access to a new medicine is initiated by a clinician at the local institution and must be approved by the hospital PTC, provincial PTC, and the NEMLC secretariat in order to be added to a tertiary EML. However, the hospital may use the medicine on a patient-named basis while awaiting the NEMLC decision.

For high cost drugs, such as biologics and oncology medicines, potential variations between facilities and provinces is further exacerbated due to a lack of consistent reviews and selection decisions. These medicines are typically approved based on a specialist's request in individual hospitals within the available budget. Although a clinical evaluation may be performed, a formal cost-effectiveness analysis is rarely ever utilized. In addition, there is limited tracking of both clinical and cost outcomes after implementation.

Reimbursement – Private Sector

In the private sector, drugs are reimbursed by the medical schemes and under Prescribed Minimum Benefits. PMBs define minimum benefits for all beneficiaries and cover nearly 270 conditions. For each condition, the minimum services level is comparable to what is provided in the public sector. While the PMB formulary may specify which class of drugs the medical schemes are required to cover, each scheme is allowed to select specific drugs within the specified classes to create its own PMB formulary. In addition, medical schemes are allowed to moderate benefits and control costs through a number of mechanisms, including established clinical protocols and formularies, preference for generics and limitations on coverage amounts.

Key mechanisms to control access to medicines in the private sector include:

1. **Formularies and clinical protocols**: medical schemes establish clinical protocols and formularies which exclude certain medications on the basis of safety and efficacy based on Health Technology Assessments (HTAs). All medicines must demonstrate that they are safe and effective, and are subject to an assessment of affordability or cost-effectiveness;

2. **Generic equivalents**: in cases where a generic equivalent has been approved for use in the medical scheme clinical protocols, funding may be capped at the price of the cheaper generic product. If a patient chooses to use the branded product over the generic, that individual would be required to pay the difference in cost via an out-of-pocket payment;

3. **Mandatory co-payment**: patients may be required to pay a mandatory co-payment of a certain amount if a medicine is approved, but perceived to be unaffordable, or if there is a supplier or market-driven demand;
4. **Capitation**: medical schemes may impose restrictions with regard to the monetary value covered, the length of treatment, or the number of treatments for a specific medicine;
5. **Self-funding gap**: in some medical schemes where patients fund medical expenses from a savings fund, exhausting available savings will result in the member falling into a self-funding gap in which the member has to cover all drugs and non-risk claims themselves. This limits the risk exposure of the medical scheme while ensuring that members are not subject to devastating financial burden as a result of medical costs.

The pathway to obtaining health technology reimbursement in the private sector in South Africa is highly formalized, with increasingly sophisticated and cost-stringent assessments by the policy units under the administration of cost-sensitive insurers. Discovery Health Medical Aid is one of the largest open medical schemes in South Africa and functions as a gatekeeper to accessing South Africa's 87 medical schemes. Other medical schemes will generally follow the findings of Discovery Health within the confines of their own scheme rules. Each medical scheme has its own process for HTAs, although none are as sophisticated as that of Discovery Health. In addition to influence on other medical schemes, reimbursement approval by Discovery Health may impact product procurement at the hospital level. Hospitals may unofficially deny their pharmacies to place a product on formulary, if it is not published on the Discovery Health Approved Product List (APL). As such, this chapter will focus on a detailed characterization of the reimbursement and HTA processes within Discovery Health as a case study for all medical schemes and a pivotal starting point for gaining access to the medical schemes in the private sector in South Africa.

As a first and largely administrative step to gaining reimbursement, manufacturers are required to apply for a National Pharmaceutical Product Index (NAPPI) code, which is crucial for insurance payers for claims purposes. The NAPPI database is a comprehensive list of pharmaceutical, surgical, and healthcare consumables products used in South Africa. Each product is allocated a unique NAPPI code which then enables providers to claim reimbursement when used. A NAPPI code application is posted to MediKredit, an independent agency responsible for the management and maintenance of the NAPPI database. However, MediKredit's role is only to correctly classify the product, not to perform any form of clinical or economic evaluation, although the assignment of a NAPPI code eventually triggers assessments by the private insurers.

Discovery Health Medical Aid—Reimbursement Evaluation Process

Clinical policy and funding decisions for medical technologies, including pharmaceuticals, devices, and procedures at Discovery Health are made via a thorough and rigorous process that involves a clinical and economic evaluation built upon the principles of evidence-based medicine and cost-effectiveness (Figure 6).

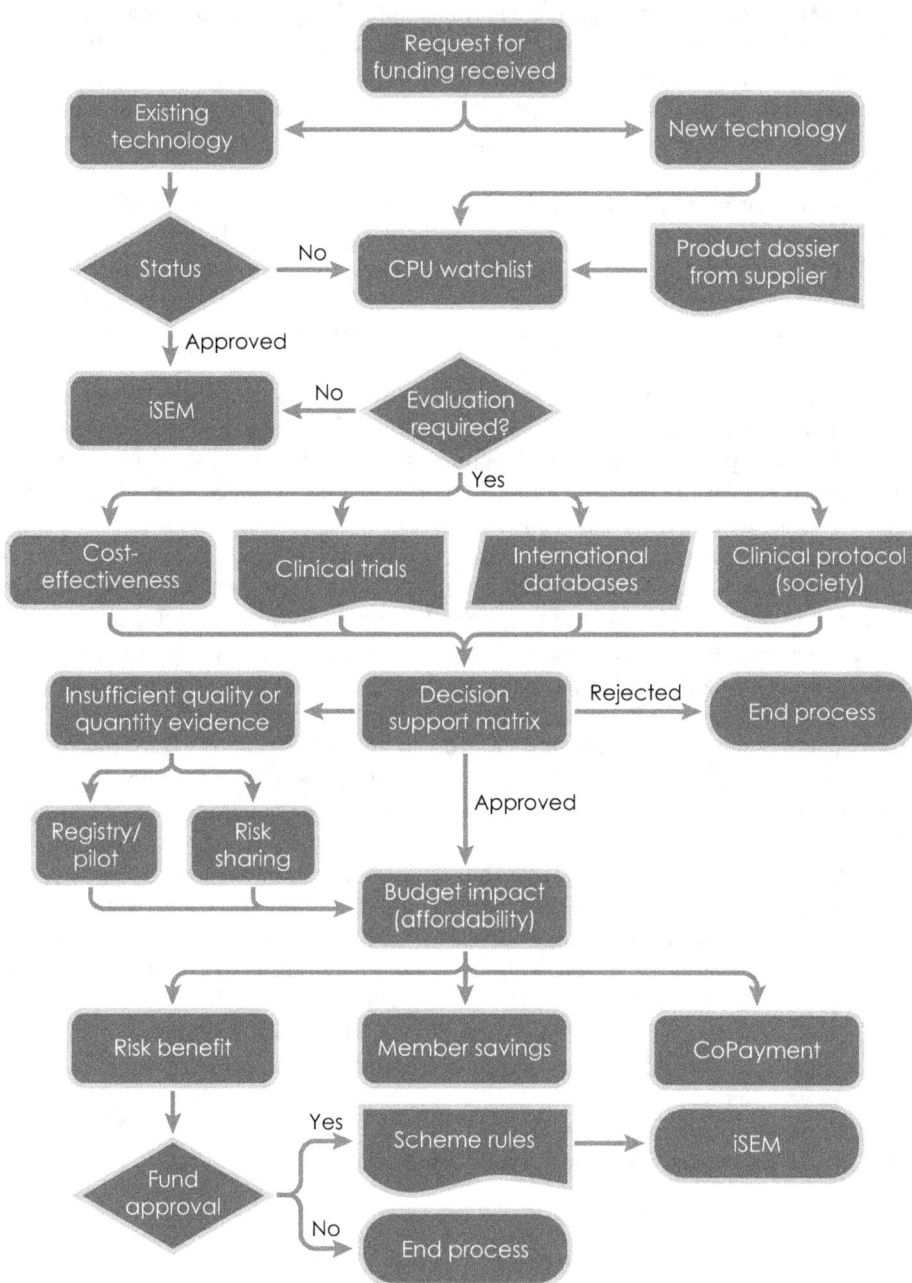

Figure 6. Discovery Health Clinical Policy and Funding Evaluation Process
CPU = Clinical Policy Unit; iSEM = in-hospital Surgical and Ethical Management

The Discovery Health reimbursement evaluation process is initiated by the in-hospital Surgical and Ethical Management (iSEM) team. New NAPPI codes automatically trigger the iSEM team to initiate the Product Introduction Notification (PIN) process, which is largely a price comparison exercise. Approval leads to the inclusion of the product onto the APL. Generally, drugs falling into an existing class or high-volume, low-cost medicines, such as statins or angiotensin-converting-enzyme (ACE) inhibitors, go through the PIN process while new and expensive technologies go straight to the Clinical Policy Unit (CPU) for a more comprehensive assessment.

The CPU within Discovery Health evaluates new, expensive technologies based on clinical safety and efficacy, cost-effectiveness and budget impact to arrive at a funding recommendation. The unit consists of an advisory board, which includes subject matter experts, clinicians, actuaries/health economists or Discovery personnel specifically trained in these areas. Applications for funding are supported by technical dossiers from manufacturers. The HTA assessment by the CPU includes an evaluation of clinical safety and effectiveness as well as cost and health economics of the new technology against the standard of care in South Africa. Discovery Health employs economic models, including both cost-effectiveness and budget impact models in order to assess affordability of the scheme. While there is no explicit threshold for cost-effectiveness, a cost per Quality-Adjusted Life Year (QALY) of three times GDP (approximately US$ 20,000 in 2013) is a common benchmark. The output of this evaluation can range from granting recommendation for approval to a conditional approval or rejection. Conditional approval is typically an outcome when a new technology is considered to have insufficient long-term data, in which case registries or pilot studies may be recommended.

Mapping and Structure of Decision Makers

The role and impact of key stakeholders in the South African market access pathways are largely understood, although nuances and complexity with regard to stakeholder interactions and influence still exist (Table 4).

One such complex relationship is the interaction among the NEMLC, provincial PTCs, and local PTCs, which varies from province to province and provides opportunities for both top-down and bottom-up influence. However, with increasing investment into the health system and a greater emphasis on more efficient provision of health services, these processes and interactions are likely to become more transparent.

As reimbursement approval processes in both the public and private sector become more established, however, opportunities for industry to directly exert influence on a funding approval process or decision is increasingly limited. Despite that, clinicians can still play a pivotal role in initiating and driving funding applications in both the public and private sector.

While both the NEMLC and provincial PTCs play a significant role in decision-making for reimbursement of drugs in the public sector, the provincial PTCs provide a greater opportunity for external influence, particularly from physicians who are able to drive funding requests at a local level. In provinces, such as Gauteng, processes have been estab-

Role	Public Sector	Private Sector
New Drug Application	Medicines Control Council (MCC)	
Formulation of health insurance and reimbursement policy	National DOH	Council for Medical Schemes (CMS)
Pricing Regulation	National DOH Tender Committee	National DOH Pricing Committee
Management of Funding/ Reimbursement	Provincial Health Departments (PHDs)	Medical Schemes
Reimbursement Application Review and Assessment	National Essential Medicines List Committee (NEMLC) for EML drugs; Provincial, District and Institutional Pharmacy and Therapeutics Committees for non-EML drugs	Medical Schemes*

Table 4. Key Stakeholders and Roles in Public and Private Market Access
CPU = Clinical Policy Unit; DOH = Department of Health; iSEM = in-hospital Surgical and Ethical Management
*Review at Discovery Health is performed by the iSEM team and CPU

lished to allow clinicians to apply for funding for new medications to be included in the EML via the provincial PTCs.

While the private sector may be fragmented across numerous medical schemes, Discovery Health remains the primary gatekeeper to private sector access and holds sway over smaller medical schemes for funding as well as procurement decisions. Medical associations and key opinion leaders (KOLs) have a voice in the CPU process and can help push for a reimbursement request, but Discovery Health is the key decision maker when it comes to obtaining reimbursement in South Africa's private sector.

Challenges and Catalyzers for Market Access

Challenges

Several key challenges exist with regard to accessing the South African market, with the key hurdles being a protracted drug registration process, lack of transparency in decision-making processes, lack of funding in the public sector, and a lack of any unified pathway to access.

The registration of pharmaceuticals under the Medicines Control Council can take on average between two to three years. This is due to a lack of sufficient resources to complete evaluations and an over-allocation of resources to the evaluation of generics. While a "fast track" process exists, this can still take 9 months and requires written notification from the Minister of Health validating that the new medicine is essential to national health. Since much of South Africa's national health focus is still on communicable diseases, such as HIV and TB, new, innovative drugs for therapeutic areas, such as oncology, continue to struggle to gain access despite the significant need for such therapies in the population.

Significant lack of transparency in the reimbursement decision-making processes also remains a key challenge, particularly with regard to inclusion on the public sector EML for reimbursement. Unlike the private sector, no formal HTA process exists in the public sector and the criteria with which new drugs are evaluated for inclusion on the EML for reimbursement is unclear.

Even if a drug is included on the EML, affordability and availability are still key barriers to the access of essential medicines. The availability of medicines is dependent on the availability of funding to each PHD and ultimately, each facility. Distribution of funding takes little account of actual activities and health needs in the country. The national government establishes allocations for the provinces and the size of conditional grants, and the provinces decide how much of their Equitable Share (ES) envelope to use on health. Distributions to the PHDs and facilities are largely historical and often insufficient.

Lastly, the lack of a unified pathway presents a challenge for manufacturers to access the South African market as a whole. While a clear division exists between the public and private sector, there is further fragmentation even within those two groups. In the public sector, the pathway and decision-making process for non-EML drugs varies from province to province, and only a few provinces have well-established drug selection processes. The Western Cape and KwaZulu-Natal have been identified as more successful examples than the other provinces in terms of drug selection.

Catalyzers

Despite these challenges, opportunities and drivers for access in South Africa still exist. Notably, South Africa serves as an entry point into the rest of Africa. Both local subsidiaries of multinational companies and South African-based distributors have long used their geographic proximity, favorable trade agreements and other historic links to export into other surrounding African Countries. Most evident of these is the SADC region, followed by COMESA and EAC, each described above. However, the Anglophone African region (ECOWAS) tends to retain its historic French distribution routes and the EAC is looking increasingly towards the East through increased trade with China and the Indian subcontinent.

Drug pricing is also relatively attractive in South Africa despite the introduction of SEP in 2006. The reason for this stems from the manner in which the industry had developed. Historically, both pharmaceuticals and medical devices had entered the market by way of local distributors. This resulted in higher consumer prices than in the product's country of origin or in other comparable markets. This entrenched, disparate pricing has continued to persist, even as local subsidiaries were established in South Africa and distributor networks were discontinued. This is particularly true for medical devices, which can be considerably more expensive in South Africa than in Western Europe. Furthermore, SEP has also virtually removed the downward pricing pressure in the private sector that is present in other markets. Since manufacturers are not allowed to sell below the SEP, their products are therefore immune to buyer pressure.

Lastly, implementation of the NHI, while still in its early stages, will have significant ramifications toward a unified pathway to access for all of South Africa. A centralized HTA process is likely to be developed as part of the NHI in order to create a united viewpoint to guide healthcare policy and coverage decisions. Several key steps have been taken towards this unified pathway, including a shift towards centralization of drug procurement and the publication of guidelines for pharmacoeconomic submissions.

7.5 Good Examples From Successful Market Access Strategies

Market access in the African region is a complex business in which language, culture, geopolitical and socioeconomic considerations influence the way products come to market and gain acceptance. The concept of reimbursement is also slightly foreign in that there is no well-established health insurance industry outside of the South African Development Community (SADC) region and products are generally purchased by healthcare providers and paid for by the government or patients. Creating relationships and networks are still central to a successful market access strategy.

Premarket approvals or regulatory access for medical products have been discussed at length for South Africa, but within the broader African continental context the situation is significantly different. Systems are generally less well-developed, but tend to cover medical devices in addition to pharmaceuticals. Furthermore, registration requirements are more pragmatic and easier to access than is the case with the MCC registration of pharmaceuticals in South Africa. However, there are various efforts underway to harmonize regulatory requirements across the region and within the trading blocs.

Historically, multinational companies have accessed the South African market by utilizing locally-based distributors and agents. Over time, these have largely been replaced by local subsidiaries of these multinational players. The distributor model is still the preferred method of entering the South African market. In the rest of Africa, the situation is similar, although there may be additional requirements for companies to have ownership vested in a citizen of the host country. This has meant there is still a greater reliance on local distributors in the rest of Africa compared to South Africa. Some multinational companies have started setting up various joint venture agreements and local ownership arrangements, which seem to be successful in facilitating local distribution.

The success of locally-based distributors and agents in Africa will be determined by the personal relationships and network of each. In East Africa, for instance, there is a significant Asian influence and distributors of this ethnic group are likely to be more successful than indigenous populations, as the main decision-makers are of Asian origin. Even within that general group, Aga Khan is the most active in the East African region which means that distributors of Ismaili origin seem to be the most successful.

Multinationals entering the African healthcare market that lack these local connections and relationships will have a more difficult route to patient access. Nevertheless, the most successful companies have been those that have invested in the development of their market. Past market development strategies have included initiating awareness campaigns, utilizing local celebrities, advertising and promotion in order to stimulate demand. These activities essentially serve to establish a market for their products where there may not have been a market previously. Diabetic products serve as a good example where this approach has been successful, as diabetes is now a key health priority for the South African government and diabetic medicines are thus well covered as part of the EML. Many of the diseases that would benefit from existing therapies go untreated. Hence, companies have to take a long-term view of the potential market and take steps to establish themselves by essentially creating the market to support their therapy.

In the South African context, the route to market is more similar to that of Western Europe and the United States. Advertising and promotion are needed to raise patient and provider awareness of available treatments as their support and pressure on funders, in particular, is important. Herceptin (trastuzumab) for treatment of breast cancer is a controversial example of the impact that public influence can have on access. The drug was evaluated by a funder and determined not to be cost-effective and therefore funding approval was denied. However, this decision was later overturned due to public and provider pressure. Regardless, any market awareness activities should be implemented as an adjunct to ensuring that all regulatory requirements are met and that each funder is proactively approached to obtain funding approval. There is no harmonized HTA process among funders or at the National or Provincial Departments of Health. Manufacturers are therefore advised to engage each potential funder individually and to ensure that they are well-aware of that funder's unique requirements. The example chosen in this chapter is Discovery Health, which appears to have the most sophisticated formalistic system of evaluation and is generally accepted as a starting point for access to the South African market. While approval by Discovery Health is not a guarantee of funding approval from other organizations, it is a strong influencing factor.

6 Outlook for the Near Future

The landscape for public healthcare funding in South Africa is expected to change radically with the institution of the NHI and the possible emergence of a national HTA agency as a potential gateway into the public sector in the future. The implementation of NHI is not only expected to impact the overall structure of the health financing system, but will also have other important ramifications for market access including harmonization of pathways, greater transparency of processes, and more efficient allocation of funding.

A proposed national HTA agency to inform NHI funding decisions will be central to the establishment of a unified pathway of market access in South Africa. The DOH is already increasingly using input from pharmacoeconomic studies to assist in reimbursement decisions. Proposals for a national HTA agency suggest modeling off Australia's Medical Services Advisory Commission (MSAC) and will take into consideration cost-effectiveness/benefit, socio/cultural/political considerations, and alternative care. Triggers for HTA will come from stakeholders and provision for stakeholder participation and transparency will be made. As such, a national HTA agency can not only provide harmonization to the fragmented market access pathways, but also increase overall transparency and opportunities for industry input in the public sector.

Furthermore, as part of the NHI, the global budget hospital payment schemes will gradually migrate towards case-based or Activity-Based Funding (ABF) under the DRGs. A DRG-based coding system is currently being developed. With the DRGs, there is expected to be a shift from historically-based budget allocations to funding based on the provision and demand of health services in each province. With more equitable distribution of funding across the provinces, there is increasing potential for more equitable access to medicines across the provinces as well.

The medical schemes in South Africa's private sector are likely to remain early opportunities for pharmaceutical companies in the near future, although several changes are underway in this industry. Escalating costs exist in private hospitals due to the fee-for-service payment system that resulted in the collapse or consolidation of many private medical schemes. For the larger schemes that remain, increasingly sophisticated HTA methodologies will be used to evaluate new therapies for reimbursement, underscoring the importance of demonstrating value of a therapy in order to successfully access the private sector.

While South Africa is one country in the diverse Sub-Saharan Africa (SSA), in many respects, South Africa could serve to be a model for other African countries in the future. Trends in harmonization of the health financing system and processes as well as the development of the private insurance system are likely to echo across the region and present opportunities in market access for SSA as a whole.

7.7 References

1. World Health Organization. Atlas of African health statistics, 2014: health situation analysis of the African region. Brazzaville, Republic of Congo: World Health Organization, Regional Office for Africa, 2014. Available at https://www.aho.afro.who.int/en/publication/921/atlas-african-health-statistics-2014-health-situation-analysis-african-region (last accessed October 2015)

2. IMS Health. Africa: A ripe Opportunity - understanding the pharmaceutical market opportunity and developing sustainable business models in Africa. London: IMS Health, 2013. Available at http://www.imshealth.com/deployedfiles/imshealth/ Global/Content/Home%20Page%20Content/High-Growth%20Markets/ Content%20Modules/IMS-Africa_WP_101212final.pdf (last accessed October 2015)

3. Ndomo A. Regional Economic Communities in Africa – A Progress Overview. Nairobi: GTZ, 2009. Available at http://www.g20dwg.org/documents/pdf/view/113 (last accessed October 2015)
4. WorldBank, 2013; http://data.worldbank.org (last accessed October 2015)
5. African Society for Laboratory Medicine. ASLM2020: Strategies and Vision to Strengthen Public Health Laboratory Medicine in Africa. Maputu: African Society for Laboratory Medicine, 2008. Available at https://www.google.it/url?sa=t&rct=j-&q=&esrc=s&source=web&cd=1&cad=rja&uact=8&ved=0CCAQFjAAahUKEwjMy8LmnerIAhWBtRQKHR5_CKI&url=https%3A%2F%2Faslm.org%2F%3Fwpdmdl%3D1&usg=AFQjCNH3nXvI0-dOgQCmwENzL6GmAaTpoA&sig2=VYfH3elSejIfJKYUqTx5Pg&bvm=bv.106379543,d.bGQ (last accessed October 2015)
6. KPMG Africa: Lifesciences. The State of Healthcare in Africa. Johannesburg: KMPG, 2012. Available at https://www.kpmg.com/Africa/en/IssuesAndInsights/Articles-Publications/Documents/The-State-of-Healthcare-in-Africa.pdf (last accessed October 2015)
7. Mostert S, Njuguna F, Olbara G, et al. Corruption in health-care systems and its effect on cancer care in Africa. *Lancet Oncol* 2015; 16: e394-e404
8. Ayodele T. Africa's Failing Approach to Health Care. National Center for Public Policy Research – A Conservative Organization, 2011. Available at https://www.nationalcenter.org/P21NVAyodeleHealth90308.html (last accessed November 2015)
9. Rispel LC, de Jager P, Fonn S. Exploring corruption in the South African health sector. Health Policy Plan 2015. pii: czv047. [Epub ahead of print]
10. WorldBank, 2011. http://www.worldbank.org (last accessed October 2015)
11. World Health Organization. South Africa: WHO statistical profile, 2015. Available at http://www.who.int/gho/countries/zaf.pdf?ua=1 (last accessed October 2015)
12. World Health Organization (2015). South Africa: Country health profile. Available at http://www.afro.who.int/en/south-africa/country-health-profile.html (last accessed October 2015)
13. National Health Act 2003, Act 61 of 2003. Available at https://www.capetown.gov.za/en/CityHealth/Documents/Legislation/Act%20-%20National%20Health%20Act%20-%2061%20of%202003.pdf (last accessed October 2015)
14. Friedrichs C. South Africa Mobile Health Market Opportunity Analysis. London: GSMA, 2012. Available at http://www.gsma.com/mobilefordevelopment/wp-content/uploads/2012/04/samobilehealthoppsfullreport.pdf (last accessed October 2015)
15. Ensor T, Kruger J, Lievens T. Improved Methods for Funding Public Hospitals in South Africa. Oxford: Oxford Policy Management, 2009. Available at http://www.opml.co.uk/sites/default/files/Financing%20hospital%20services%20in%20South%20Africa%20021209_0.pdf (last accessed October 2015)
16. McLeod H. (2012). HMR-SEPOCT 2012: Executive Summary of Policy Brief – NHI Pilot Sites. Hanmer Springs: IMSA, 2010. Available at http://www.edoc.co.za/modules.php?name=News&file=article&sid=4290 (last accessed October 2015)

17. CMS. Council for Medical Schemes Annual Report 2013/2014. Pretoria: CMS, 2014. Available at https://www.medicalschemes.com/files/Annual%20Reports/AR2013_2014LR.pdf (last accessed October 2015)

18. Ruff P. Regulation and Funding of Medicines in South Africa, 2015. Available at https://am.asco.org/regulation-and-funding-medicines-south-africa (last accessed October 2015)

19. Gray AL. Medicine Pricing Interventions – the South African experience. Available at http://apps.who.int/medicinedocs/documents/s16379e/s16379e.pdf (last accessed October 2015)

20. Department of Health. Registration of Medicines – General Information. Pretoria, 2012: MCC. Available at https://www.google.it/url?sa=t&rct=j&q=&esrc=s&source=web&cd=1&ved=0CCAQFjAAahUKEwjYg-uT-fHIAhVDig8KHUC7At8&url=http%3A%2F%2Fwww.rrfa.co.za%2Fwp-content%2Fuploads%2F2012%2F11%2F2.01_General_information_Jul12_v8_showing_changes.docx&usg=AFQjCNHxs53o8W_uEIgvxlVqgni5sbIQYw&sig2=5IEDwK4wh-imtF0PNk5Z0A&bvm=bv.106379543,d.bGQ&cad=rja (last accessed November 2015)

21. IMS Institute for Healthcare Informatics (2015). Understanding the Role and Use of Essential Medicines Lists. London: IMS Health, 2015. Available at https://www.imshealth.com/imshealth/Global/Content/Corporate/IMS%20Health%20Institute/Insights/IIHI_Essential_Medicines_Report_2015.pdf (last accessed October 2015)

22. Lymphoma Coalition. (2013). South Africa Drug Funding/Reimbursement Approval Process. Available at http://www.lymphomacoalition.org/docman2/leip-reports/leip-2013/356-south-africa-funding-process-flowchart-october-2013 (last accessed October 2015)

23. Gauteng Province Health. Gauteng Provincial Pharmacy and Therapeutics Committee – Biennial Report 1 April 2012 – 31 March 2014. 2015. Available at http://siapsprogram.org/publication/gauteng-provincial-pharmacy-and-therapeutics-committee-biennial-report-1-april-2012-31-march-2014/ (last accessed October 2015)

7.8 To know more

- African Society for Laboratory Medicine. Ministerial Call for Action - Strengthening Laboratory Services in Africa. Cape Town: ASLM, 2014
- Azatyan S. Overview of African Medicines Registration Harmonization Initiative (AMRH). Ottawa: VII Conference of the Pan American Network on Drug Regulatory Harmonization (PANDRH), 2013. Available at https://www.google.it/url?sa=t&rct=j&q=&esrc=s&source=web&cd=1&ved=0CCAQFjAAahUKEwjE8dDzsurIAhVCRhQKHRPcA-0&url=http%3A%2F%2Fwww.paho.org%2Fhq%2Findex.php%3Foption%3Dcom_docman%26task%3Ddoc_download%26gid%3D22866%

26Itemid%3D270%26lang%3Dpt&usg=AFQjCNHf4BMy70Su_6lgk4w8C6Zf-Yt9 LA&sig2=AU4o2dMjDCq3RMjVbUI2iA&bvm=bv.106379543,d.bGQ&cad=rja (last accessed October 2015)

- Buch E, Hogerzeil H. African Medicines Registration Harmonisation (AMRH) Initiative: Summary, Status and Future Plans. Johannesburg: The New Partnership for Africa's Development (NEPAD) & the World Health Organization (WHO), 2009. Available at http://apps.who.int/medicinedocs/documents/s20130en/s20130en. pdf (last accessed October 2015)
- Byl S, Punia M, Owino R. Devolution of Healthcare Services in Kenya. Johannesburg: KPMG, 2013. Available at https://www.kpmg.com/Africa/en/ IssuesAndInsights/Articles-Publications/Documents/Devolution%20of%20 HC%20Services%20in%20Kenya.pdf (last accessed October 2015)
- Deloitte Touche Tohmastsu Ltd. Insights into the high-level financial contribution of the Pharmaceutical Industry in South Africa. Johannesburg: Deloitte Touche Tohmastsu Ltd, 2010. Available at http://s3.amazonaws.com/zanran_storage/ www.imsa.org.za/ContentPages/2470361400.pdf (last accessed October 2015)
- Department of Health. Annual Report 2013-2014. Pretoria: Government Publisher, 2014. Available at http://www.gov.za/sites/www.gov.za/files/Department_of_ Health_Annual_Report_2014.pdf (last accessed November 2015)
- Department of Health. SA Yearbook 2013/2014. Pretoria: GCIS, 2014. Available at http://www.gcis.gov.za/content/resourcecentre/sa-info/yearbook2013-14 (last accessed November 2015)
- Directorate of Registration and Regulatory Affairs. Guidelines for Registration of Imported Drug Products in Nigeria (NAFDAC/RR/002/00). Available at Lagos: NAFDAC, 2000. http://apps.who.int/medicinedocs/documents/s17115e/s17115e. pdf (last accessed November 2015)
- Department of Trade and Industry. Department of Trade and Industry Import Trade Statistics. Pretoria: DTI, 2014. Available at http://tradestats.thedti.gov. za/ReportFolders/reportFolders.aspx?sCS_referer=&sCS_ChosenLang=en (last accessed November 2015)
- Health Systems Trust. South African Health Review. Durban: Health Systems Trust, 2013. Available at http://www.hst.org.za/sites/default/files/SAHR2012_13_ lowres_1.pdf (last accessed November 2015)
- Health Systems Trust. Health Statistics. 2015. Available at http://indicators.hst. org.za/healthstats/112/data (last accessed November 2015)
- Hodge J, Fiandeiro F, Lynch S, et al. 2015. Background Papers and Studies. Available at http://www.compcom.co.za/healthcare-market-background-papers/ (last accessed November 2015)
- Insight Actuaries and Consultants. International Benchmarking of Hospital Utilization: How does South African Private Hospital Sector Compare? Johannesburg: Hospital Association of South Africa, 2014. Available at http://www.hasa.co.za/wp-content/ uploads/2015/02/HASA-Intl-utilisation-benchmarking-Final-201411231-copy1.pdf (last accessed November 2015)

- Kenya Pharmacy Poisons Board. Guidelines on Submission of Documentation for Registration of Medical Devices. Nairobi: KPPB, 2011. Available at https://www.google.it/url?sa=t&rct=j&q=&esrc=s&source=web&cd=1&ved=0CCA QFjAAahUKEwi1wPix5vHIAhVEJA8KHaSRAds&url=http%3A%2F%2Fpharmacyb oardkenya.org%2Fdownloads%2F%3Ffile%3Dmedical_devices_guidelines.pdf&usg =AFQjCNGE40wzU5WgpVSkYK8GaqGu0AtjCw&sig2=FRqF1nif86uxhMYQF0Dx0 A&cad=rja (last accessed November 2015)
- Life Healthcare. 2015. Company Overview. http://lifehealthcare.co.za/Company/Default.aspx (last accessed November 2015)
- McKinsey & Company. A view on Medical Devices in Africa. Presented at Euro-Africa Health Investment Conference. McKinsey and Company, 2013. Available at http://www.slideshare.net/PharmaAfrica/a-view-on-medical-devices-in-africa (last accessed November 2015)
- Mediclinic. 2015. About us. Available at http://www.mediclinic.co.za/about/Pages/default.aspx (last accessed November 2015)
- Medikredit. 2015. NAPPI Product Search Facility. Retrieved from Medikredit: https://www.medikredit.co.za/index.php?option=com_nappi&Itemid=210 (last accessed November 2015)
- Medpages. 2015. Medical professionals healthcare professionals in South Africa: 29 Jun 2015. Available at: http://www.medpages.co.za/sf/index.php?page=categoryst ats&countryid=1&categoryid=1 (last accessed October 2015)
- Musango L, Elovainio R, Nabyonga J, et al. The state of health financing in the African Region. *African Health Monitor* 2016; 16: 9-14. Available at http://www.aho.afro.who.int/sites/default/files/ahm/reports/556/ahm1603.pdf (last accessed November 2015)
- NAFDAC. Automated Product Administration and Monitoring System. Lagos: NAFDAC, 2010
- National Department of Health. 2012. Regulations relating to Categories of Hospitals R185. *Government Gazette No 35101*. Pretoria, Gauteng, South Africa: Government Gazette.
- Netcare. 2015. Netcare. http://www.netcareinvestor.co.za/over_structure.php (last accessed November 2015)
- African Society for Laboratory Medicine. EAC Progress Towards Harmonizing The Regulation Of Diagnostics in The EAC. ASLM First International Conference. Cape Town, 2012
- Olugbenga EO. The Politics of Pharmaceutical Regulation in Nigeria: Policy Options for Third World Countries. *Public Policy and Administration Research* 2013; 3: 89-101. Available at http://www.iiste.org/Journals/index.php/PPAR/article/view/7105/7338 (last accessed November 2015)
- Pillay A. Medicine price regulation – the South African experience. Available at http://www.ipc-undp.org/pressroom/files/ipc144.pdf (last accessed November 2015)

- Pharmacy and Poisons Board. Registration of Drugs: Guidelines to Submission of Applications. Nairobi: PPB, 2010. Available at http://apps.who.int/medicinedocs/documents/s21380en/s21380en.pdf (last accessed November 2015)
- Shabangu T. Country Data Profile on the Pharmaceutical Situation in the Southern African Development Community (SADC). Pretoria, 2009: WHO. Available at http://apps.who.int/medicinedocs/documents/s17215e/s17215e.pdf (last accessed November 2015)
- Shunmugam, V. (2015, 5 18). Written Feedback to Survey Questions for Mediclinic (M. Banfield, Interviewer)
- Stander MP, Bergh M, Miller-Jansön HE. A first step towards transparency in pricing of medicines and scheduled substances - publication of guidelines for pharmaco-economic submissions. *S Afr Med J* 2013; 104: 10-1
- Stats SA. General Household Survey. Pretoria: Stats SA, 2014. Available at http://www.statssa.gov.za/publications/P0318/P03182013.pdf (last accessed November 2015)
- Stats SA. Use of health facilities and levels of selected health conditions in South Africa: Findings from the General Household Survey. Pretoria: Stats SA, 2011. Available at http://www.statssa.gov.za/publications/Report-03-00-05/Report-03-00-052011.pdf (last accessed November 2015)
- Strachan B, Zabow T, vanderSpuy Z. More doctors and dentists are needed in South Africa. *S Afr Med J* 2011; 101: 523-8
- Stirling C. More Than Medicine. Johannesburg: KPMG, 2013. Available at https://www.kpmg.com/Global/en/IssuesAndInsights/ArticlesPublications/more-than-medicine/Documents/more-than-medicine-v1.pdf (last accessed November 2015)
- Briggs J. The Processes and Requirements for the Introduction of Combination Therapy in Selected African Countries. United States Agency for International Development, 2002. Available at http://pdf.usaid.gov/pdf_docs/Pnadl909.pdf (last accessed November 2015)
- van den Heever, A. Review of Competition in the South African Healthcare System. Pretoria: Competition Commission, 2015
- van Rooyen, H. (2015, 5 19). Written response to survey questionnaire (M. Banfield, Interviewer)
- Wamae W, Kungu JK, Clark N, et al. Spotlight on pharmaceutical pricing regulation in Kenya: how much does it really contribute to access? African Centre for Technology Studies, 2014. Available at http://iphsp.acts-net.org/images/briefs/Pricing-brief.pdf (last accessed November 2015)
- WESGRO. WESGRO Research Report Sector Medical Devices. Cape Town: WESGRO, 2014. Available at http://wesgro.co.za/publications/publication/2014-western-cape-medical-devices-sector (last accessed November 2015)
- Wilsdon T, Fiz E, Haderi A. A comparative analysis of the role and impact of Health Technology Assessment: 2013. London, 2014: Charles River Associates. Available

at http://www.efpia.eu/uploads/documents/cra-comparative-analysis.pdf (last accessed November 2015)

- World Health Organization. World Health Statistics 2006 – Table 6. Geneva, 2006: WHO. Available at http://www.who.int/gho/publications/world_health_statistics/whostat2006_erratareduce.pdf (last accessed November 2015)
- World Health Organization. Assessment of medicines regulatory systems in Sub-Saharan African Countries. Geneva, 2010: WHO. Available at http://apps.who.int/medicinedocs/documents/s17577en/s17577en.pdf (last accessed November 2015)
- World Health Organization. *Health Systems Financing – The path to universal coverage.* Geneva, 2010: WHO. Available at http://www.who.int/whr/2010/10_summary_en.pdf (last accessed November 2015)
- World Health Organization. *Nigeria Pharmaceutical Country Profile.* Lagos, 2011: Federal Ministry of Health in collaboration with the WHO. Available at http://www.who.int/medicines/areas/coordination/Nigeria_PSCPNarrativeQuestionnaire_01062011.pdf (last accessed November 2015)
- World Health Organization. Noncommunicable Diseases (NCD) Country Profiles. Geneva, 2014: WHO. Available at http://www.who.int/nmh/countries/zaf_en.pdf?ua=1 (last accessed November 2015)

Market Access in Turkey

Fatma Betul Yenilmez
With the collaboration of Güvenç Koçkaya

General Overview of Healthcare System and Health Policies

In 2003, the Health Transformation Program (HTP) was implemented to reduce inequities in health financing, health service access, and outcomes [1], and Social Security reform followed in 2006 due to the need for sustainability [2].

The health insurance system in Turkey (Figure 1) before 2006 was a combined model, but the current Social Security system is based on premiums (Beveridge model). With Social Security reform, the government should contribute 20% of the premiums collected and pays premiums instead of the poors. Under this system, the employers' share of civil servants' social security premiums are financed from the government budget, specifically by taxes. In other words, the government implemented a premium system for the poor and civil servants instead of paying healthcare expenditures indirectly by taxes, as was done prior to Social Security reform.

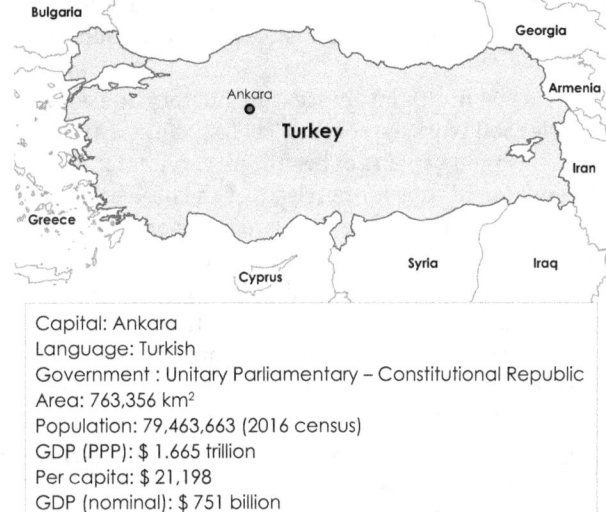

Capital: Ankara
Language: Turkish
Government : Unitary Parliamentary – Constitutional Republic
Area: 763,356 km²
Population: 79,463,663 (2016 census)
GDP (PPP): $ 1.665 trillion
Per capita: $ 21,198
GDP (nominal): $ 751 billion
Per capita: $ 9,562
Currency: Turkish Lira (TL)

Figure 1. Turkey: map and features

Social Security reform has gathered the four major plans of the health insurance system under a single roof. As a result, the Social Security Institution [3] (SGK) has become the largest payer for healthcare services in Turkey since 2008.

The Ministry of Health (MoH) is the health authority in Turkey, while the Turkish Medicines and Medical Devices Agency (TITCK) [4] is the agency responsible for the pharmaceutical and medical devices sectors on behalf of the MoH. The function of TITCK is licensing, auditing, and also regulating the pharmaceutical sector, pharmacies, and the medical devices market.

In the pharmaceutical sector, there are over 24,000 pharmacies operating in Turkey. Every pharmacy should be owned and operated by a pharmacist. Indeed, pharmacy chains or pharmacy ownership by any party other than a pharmacist is not allowed in Turkey.

All pharmaceutical products should be licensed and priced by the MoH in order to attend to the market in Turkey. The MoH controls the pharmaceutical and medical devices market and public hospitals via the Turkish Public Hospital Union Agency [5]. TITCK determines the clinical approvals of clinical trial, licensing, and pricing of pharmaceuticals and cosmetics, the running of the Pharmaceuticals Electronic Tracking System (ITS) [6], the registration of medical devices, the operation of the pharmacovigilance system, the assessment of applications for off-label medicine use, and so on. The agency is also responsible for market supervision and the surveillance of medicines.

Universal health insurance is mandatory and covers all the insured population under a single roof. Workers, soldiers, civil servants, artisans, and the poor are all subject to the same rules and benefits of healthcare services. The SGK serves over 85% of the total population [7] and pays for nearly all of the healthcare services in Turkey. The benefit package is wide, and there are only two levels of contribution – 10% for pensioners and 20% for active employees (same for dependents) – for pharmaceuticals. Nearly all pharmaceuticals for chronic disease and life threatening conditions are fully reimbursed. Moreover, medical examinations and pharmaceuticals for most chronic diseases and life threatening conditions are exempted from contribution for all users.

There are both international and local companies present in the pharmaceutical market in Turkey. The international companies have a lower share in terms of volume but a higher share in overall value (Turkish Lira – TL); conversely, the local companies has just the opposite. International companies mainly have patented products; on the other hand, local companies have mainly generics on the market.

8.2 Pathways of Market Access (Regulation, Pricing, and Reimbursement)

The MoH does not heavily regulate healthcare interventions, generally leaving the practice up to clinicians. However, the pharmaceutical area is strictly regulated in Turkey, as it is in the rest of the world. In this section, details will be provided about the legal procedures related to pharmaceuticals.

Pharmaceutical Licensing

The Turkish Medicines and Medical Devices Agency, a related institution of the MoH, is the licensing authority for pharmaceuticals. Local clinical data is not mandatory, which means that clinical data can be obtained worldwide. The Turkish Medicines and Medical Devices Agency accepts pharmaceutical licensing approvals in Common Technical Document (CTD) format. The agency staff then verifies the contents of the documents.

There is a Licensing Committee that advises the Agency about licensing approvals. The Committee is composed of part-time academics from University Hospitals. Sub-committees can be created to work in more detail. The Licensing Committee consults on the dossier and advises the Agency. However, the TITCK makes decisions independently of the European Medicines Agency (EMA). In addition, both the Agency and Licensing Committee consider Food and Drug Agency (FDA) from United States or European Medicines Agency (EMA) from European Union approvals. The context of such approvals may be as broad or tighter than EMA or FDA decisions.

The Good Manufacturing Practice (GMP) Audit was legally regulated before the Agency began to put it into practice in March 2010. Since then, a GMP audit has become mandatory for licensing both for manufactured and imported pharmaceuticals. It does not matter, however, whether or not the FDA and/or EMA license the manufacturer. The bioequivalence regulations for generics were went in to effect in May 1994 and came into practice over a five-year period, following the patent law for pharmaceuticals that was implemented in 1999 by decree number 566.

Pharmaceuticals Pricing

The TITCK is the pricing authority for pharmaceuticals also. An international reference pricing system was implemented due to the Council of Ministers Decree in 2005. While several updates have been made to the processes and rates, the reference countries remain the same: France, Portugal, Spain, Italy, and Greece are the main reference countries for all pharmaceuticals. In these reference countries, the license holder company should submit the ex-factory price of the pharmaceutical product. Moreover, the manufacturing country of origin and the import country prices should be submitted if there is any change from the main reference countries.

The main exchange currency is the Euro. To prevent price fluctuations due to currency changes, the annual weighted average previous year currency rate announced by the Central Bank of Turkey with a 30% discount is taken into account to calculate the prices for the following year.

Original and generic products can be priced at 100% or 60% of calculated ex-factory price with given reference price and fixed exchange rate, respectively. There is a group of pharmaceuticals referred to as "20-year medicine" in Turkey. When implementing the international reference price system in 2005, the very old medicines (those licensed anywhere throughout the world before 1985, meaning 20 years or less) were exempted so as not to cause very low and unsustainable prices. The exemption date of origin was updated only once and defined as the molecules licensed anywhere in the world before 1987 (this is still in effect). This group was exempted from international reference pricing before 2010, but by that time the ones more expensive than 10 TL were also required to declare the reference prices.

There are some exemptions in pricing procedures and rates for blood products, nutritional products, radio pharmaceuticals, etc. In addition, orphan drugs are not well defined, and the pricing procedure for them is the same as for other pharmaceuticals.

International reference pricing refers to the ex-factory price. The TITCK announces the market price, adding on wholesaler and pharmacy margins, both of which are progressively calculated, and 8% VAT over the ex-factory price. The margins of wholesalers and pharmacies vary depending on the calculated Turkish Lira ex-factory price.

Pharmaceutical Reimbursement

The SGK, an institution related to the Ministry of Labor and Social Security (MoL&SS), is the reimbursement authority for pharmaceuticals.

In 2006, with the Social Security reform, a positive list of products was composed. All the products in the market are added to the list, which means that the products are not assessed individually. After the list was formed, licensed products were obligated to apply according to the Directive of Working Procedures and Principles of the Reimbursement Commission [9]; further, a Drug Application Instruction was announced along with the Directive.

Companies need to apply to the SGK according to the Directive and Instructions after receiving a license and price from the MoH-TITCK for pharmaceuticals. Only prescription drugs can be reimbursed, although blood products, nutritional products, radiation medicines, and medicines brought from abroad with TITCK approval are also reimbursable.

Pharmaceutical companies should apply with a reimbursement dossier including a cost-effectiveness and budget impact analysis with a three-year time frame and payer perspective to SGK, prepared according to the Directive and Instructions. Cost-utility analysis are not acceptable for the application.

The Drug Application Instructions contain a detailed list of required documents. First, the applications need to be discussed by a technical commission. This is coordinated by the SGK Directorate General of Universal Health Insurance with representatives of the SGK, TITCK, Ministry of Finance, Ministry of Development, Undersecretary of Treasure, and pharmaceutical associations. Unfortunately, there is no defined representation from patient or health professional organizations. The committee frequently requests the opinions of clinicians from medical associations interested in related topics. The companies are informed in the event of refusal; the reimbursement decisions are announced in an official gazette and/or the web site of the Institution.

8.3 Mapping and Structure of Decision-Makers

The main decision-makers in the healthcare and pharmaceutical markets are governmental organizations. There is a huge Social Security system and public administration of most healthcare providers.

The MoH is one of the most important stakeholders because it is the health authority as well as the largest health care provider; the Ministry of Labor and Social Security (MoL&SS) is another important stakeholder because it is almost the single payer. Today, private health insurance covers approximately three million people.

The Ministry of Finance, Ministry of Development, and Undersecretary of Treasury are other important stakeholders, especially in regard to reimbursement procedures and the planning of health policy.

Turkey is aware of the need to conduct a Health Technology Assessment (HTA) to assess health technologies and attempt to improve their capacity. There are three different governmental HTA bodies formed in Turkey:

- The first is the TITCK, which is related to the MoH, has a basic interest in health policy issues, and published one report by the end of 2014;
- The second is under the Directorate General for Health Research, which is related to the MoH and has published four reports about clinical processes [7];
- The third is a part of the reimbursement authority SSI, related to the MoL&SS; unfortunately, it has published no reports to date;

There is also a local HTA body that operates as part of a third-tier public hospital. Its reports can be found at http://hta.gov.tr/raporlar.aspx.

The physician organizations affect decision-makers through the committees that advise authorities, but unfortunately the patient organizations are weak. In fact, both physicians and patients can affect and change the unappropriated decree for them judicially.

4   Challenges and Catalysts for Market Access

Challenges

The delayed market access timeline due to GMP auditing, licensing, and reimbursement appears to be the most important challenge for pharmaceutical market access in Turkey. After implementing the common positive list in 2006, which required that every new product be assessed prior to reimbursement, decisions on reimbursement seem to have delayed entering the market. In addition, patient-specific procurement from abroad under off-licence became an important access channel in this period.

The GMP audit procedure is the most important contributor to delayed market access in recent years. The Association of Research-Based Pharmaceutical Companies (AIFD) has published several reports to show the effect of GMP audits on delayed market access. According to their last Inquiry Report, physical inspection took an average of 476 days for inspected products, and more than half of the applications had already been waiting for an average of 548 days [8].

There are three national and one local HTA body working in Turkey, but their positions on procedures are not well defined. Moreover, the national HTA department of the MoH can affect reimbursement decisions with its published reports. Unfortunately, the technical capacity of the HTA bodies is not sufficient.

Another policy tool that represents a huge challenge for pharmaceuticals is the government's forcing down of prices in Turkey. The exchange currency rate is fixed and the single payer SGK requires additional high discount rates in order to get reimbursement.

Both the low price policy and single payer situation have negative secondary effects globally and locally. For example, the low price policy threatens sustainable global prices because some other countries refer to Turkey for international reference pricing. Locally, because of the national reimbursement agency, none of the pharmaceuticals can survive outside of the "single" positive list.

Catalysts

The nationwide reimbursement agency presents a significant challenge but also provides an opportunity to access the market. Unlike most other countries such as Spain or the USA, the companies in Turkey must struggle and pay only one institution. Turkey has a huge population, over 78 million in 2015, all of which is under a single insurance plan. When a pharmaceutical company decides to enter the Turkish market and is reimbursed for its products, everyone in the country has the opportunity to get those products. Thus, when a company is added to the positive list, it has the chance to sell to a population that is larger than that of most European countries.

8.5 Good Examples from Successful Market Access Strategies

The main stakeholders believe that Turkey offers a large market for pharmaceuticals and has a large budget for healthcare facilities. The share of pharmaceutical expenditures comprises over 30% of the total health care expenditures. This has the potential of grooving due to increased access to healthcare and the population aging forecast. In the short term, decision-makers have decided to manage the expenditures by regulating pricing and reimbursement. However, some different tools have been implemented to promote the manufacturing of pharmaceuticals locally in Turkey.

Good Manufacturing Practice (GMP) Audit

The national GMP audit capacity is just growing and is not yet sufficient to meet the country's need. The authority (TITCK) is planning to request GMP audits according to the needs of Turkish patients, the national prioritization, and emergency requirements, within the boundaries of institutional capability. As a result of the increasing discussions on the quality of healthcare services and pharmaceuticals, the whole healthcare system in Turkey is in need of tools of increasing quality. At this point, the GMP audit practice allows the pharmaceutical market to declare its quality of manufacturing. Healthcare providers such as hospitals or medical device suppliers still need to prove the quality of their services.

Promoting Generics

Local manufacturers are basically marketing generics. Two-thirds of units of consumed medicines belongs to these manufacturers, but they only get one-third of the budget. The original and generics all have brand names in Turkey, and they are all set in the same internal reference pricing basket during reimbursement.

Another point is that "local manufactured" products seem to be promoted, but the concept of "locak manufactured" is not well defined. It is not clear if "locally manufactured" means that all production stages occur locally in Turkey or if simply pressing tablets or fill and finish are also accepted as manufacturing. Unfortunately, no clear differentiation has yet been made.

.6 Look-up for Near Future

The national medicine policy for managing pharmaceutical expenditures has been based on "price" since 2005. Initially (from 2005 to 2009), the main mechanism was controlling the market price; then beside it, the reimbursement price from 2010 to 2012. In the same period, a "prescription fee" was initiated to control the demand side. For the updated information, the tools are reference pricing, the exchange rate for official price, and discount rates for reimbursement.

The government stakeholders are aware of the descending profit margins on pharmaceutical prices and the increasing share of out-of-pocket payment; one cause is the companies and the other is that the beneficiaries are not satisfied. Hence, policymakers are discussing alternative tools that they could use to manage pharmaceutical expenditures.

Market Access Agreements could be applied primarily to the pharmaceuticals that may have a high budget impact. The Social Security Institution initiated a directive called "Working Principles of the Commission of Alternative Reimbursement Procedures for Health Care Services" on April 30, 2015. In addition, the Drug Reimbursement Principles and Procedures of Their Application was announced on March 2016. These legislations are aimed at the implementation of Market Access Agreements (local defined as Alternative Reimbursement Regulations) in Turkey. After the establishment of new legislation, some innovative pharmaceuticals received reimbursements with Market Access Agreements on June 2016. Depending on best knowledge, Market Access Agreements are based on financial rather than performance-based circumstances. Market access agreements will be one of important key tool for pharmaceutical market access in Turkey for near future.

8.7 References

1. Atun R, Aydın S, Chakraborty S, et al. Universal health coverage in Turkey: enhancement of equity. *Lancet* 2013; 382: 65-99
2. Alper Y. Reform in the Turkish social security system and expectations about financing. *Journal of Social Security (Sosyal Güvenlik Dergisi)* 2012; 1: 7-47
3. Social Security Institution – SGK (*Sosyal Güvenlik Kurumu*). Available at http://www.sgk.gov.tr/wps/portal/sgk/en/home-page/mainpage (last accessed September 2016)
4. Turkish Medicines and Medical Device Agency – TITCK (*Türkiye İlaç ve Tıbbi Cihaz Kurumu*). Available at http://www.titck.gov.tr (last accessed September 2016)
5. Turkish Public Hospital Union Agency – TKHK (*Türkiye Kamu Hastaneleri Kurumu*). Available http://www.tkhk.gov.tr (last accessed September 2016)
6. Electronic Tracking System – ITS (*İlaç Takip Sistemi*). Available at http://itsportal. saglik.gov.tr (last accessed September 2016)
7. General Directorate of Health Researches – SAGEM. Available at http://hta.gov.tr/ raporlar.aspx (last accessed September 2016)
8. Association of Research-Based Pharmaceutical Companies – AiFD (*Arastirmaci Ilac Firmalari Dernegi*). Available at http://www.aifd.org.tr/ (last accessed September 2016)

Comparing the Market Access and HTA process of Selected Countries from Different Regions

Mete Saylan, Özge Dokuyucu

Introduction

Real applications and the concept of "Health Technology Assessment (HTA)" surged in the beginning of the 1980s due to inevitable growth of innovative health technologies and limited health budgets of governments. The HTA agencies involve different disciplines and stakeholders. Generally HTA is used as an input to the reimbursement decisions, which may affect positively or negatively on patient's access to medicines. Although HTA is used as a tool to allocate optimal resources, it may delay patient's access to new drugs as it is designed to be an additional step prior launch in many countries.

Stakeholders can be defined based on influencers and influenced groups within the whole process of HTA. The HTA agencies generally utilize comprehensive data sets and gather different stakeholders including, healthcare professionals and academicians from research institutes, healthcare providers, health policy decision makers and their officers. The effect size of HTA agencies can be as narrow as a treatment protocol in a single clinic or it can be very broad to set priorities and to make decisions within the healthcare systems. However, HTA is not the sole component of the inputs used for decision making and its relative role changes depending on the position of other components within a healthcare system.

In a broad sense, HTA can be defined as a tool used by decision makers and advisors between decision making and research domains. It includes analysis of different overlapping areas (technology, the patients, the organization and the economy) where the research questions have important health consequences. With the development of "the evidence based healthcare system" concept in 1990s, evidence became the key common element of HTA. Even though HTA is for practical use in different systems, HTA has to be based on universal scientific methods. The organizational basis of HTA agencies may have a decisive influence on the target groups. Depending on organizational basis, target groups may be small (management of a specific clinic) or larger (regional administrators, Ministry of Health, funding institutions). Specific principles were designed by international academicians and leaders to guide the conduct and evaluation of HTA. The intended audiences of the principles include those working in HTA as well as all decision makers, including patients. Their aim is to improve the concepts and practice of HTA. However, their studies demonstrated considerable variation in uptake of the principles [1].

9.2 Comparing HTA systems

Despite similarities in the HTA related question(s) for the same decision making process and efforts to internationalize it, the HTA of each system, by nature, becomes unique. Therefore, comparative assessment of HTA systems emerges unavoidably in the minds in order to designate best practices from different national models in the world. Various published studies have already compared HTA systems from different perspectives and they tried to find the best way to perform HTA [1-4]. Our aim is to compare different HTA from scope and perspective, process and methodology, impact and outcome, as well as quality perspectives and to elucidate differences that originate from the structure of their respective health system. In Table 1 is reported the comparative assessment methodology.

There is widely available literature on the proposed best methodologies for conducting HTA assessment [5-7]. Different agencies are involved in different countries with different standpoints in terms of health policy. However, there are also counties which do not have a specific HTA agency with specified guidance on undertaking assessments. We have selected a number of countries that may represent the overall picture.

Scope and perspective

HTA scope and perspective feeds into pricing and reimbursement in many markets; some are more clearly defined as they use clinically measured added benefit (e.g. ASMR rating in France) or by setting a threshold to measure a product's cost-effectiveness. Practices about the inclusion of societal value within the full assessment are diversified. However, in many countries where societal value is included in the assessment it is considerably less impactful on decision making. Innovative drug companies can communicate with the HTA agency at the early development stage which enables to clarify the assessment process and requirements they will be asked to fulfill. Uncertainty of HTA findings is a growing concern among payers and many of them try to minimize it by developing

Scope and perspective	Process and methodology	Impact and outcome	Quality
• Clear HTA objective of use • Restriction of new technologies • Openness with industry when setting the scope • Management of uncertainty	• Limiting by delayed review timelines • Setting clear requirements • Involvement of all stakeholders	• Impact on society • Local setting adjustment • Taking responsibility of the outcome	• Use of comprehensive data set • Qualified and adequate human resources

Table 1. Comparative Assessment Methodology

structured processes. Countries with more formal assessment process reports explicitly the degree of uncertainties to highlight its role in the decision making. Consequently, in many countries different types of risk sharing agreements are used to address uncertainties.

Process and methodology

The methods and approach used by HTA agencies as a guideline documented in their websites. Others provided documentations about the approach used but they are not clearly defined or they are not strictly followed in practice. In countries where HTA is still under development, the evaluation method and processes are relatively less transparent. Although it's a common view of the all HTA reviews that the involvement of all potential stakeholders is the key for a successful HTA, the role of other stakeholders (e.g. patient groups) stayed very limited. A majority of the agencies did not state their goal for duration of reviews. Actual median time to review or to decision is available from case studies or industry reports. It's not possible to compare directly median times to decision because reviews can begin before a product is approved or product is reimbursed prior to decision in many markets as an effort to reduce delays in market access. In general, the length of the time between marketing authorization and reimbursement decision varies by products and the lengths of reviews differ among different HTA agencies.

Impact and outcome

The impact of HTA findings are monitored in some countries by a responsible body to evaluate whether its results are incorporated to process, as well as the decision is re-evaluated by collecting data to measure its clinical impact over time. Reviews of the impact of different HTA on a group of medical technologies in a specified time frame can be used as a proxy to understand the impact of these evaluations on price, timing, reimbursement and restrictions enforced on technologies. The relationship between price, reimbursement restrictions and rewarding value is less clear in many of these systems. In many of them findings of HTA are not followed during the decision of pricing and reimbursement bodies. There is also significant variation in the restrictions applied for the same products as a result of the similar HTA results. We observed that in countries where the impact of HTA is monitored, there is also a process to improve the quality of outcomes over time.

Quality

Governments, the main founders of HTA agencies were challenged by the scarcity of resources problem for the growing number of reviews needed to be completed within the limited time frame. This is mostly valid for relatively new HTA agencies where trained HTA evaluators are very limited. Budget, human resources, availability of local data and usability of results by the health system often determine the quality of the assessment.

Country	HTA Agency	Scope and Perspective	Process and Methodology	Impact and Outcome	Quality
Australia	PBAC	+++	+++	+++	+++
Brazil	CITEC	+	+	+	+
Canada	CADTH	++	+++	+++	+++
England	NICE	+++	+++	+++	+++
France	HAS (CT)	+++	++	+++	+++
Germany	IQWIG	++	++	+	+++
Israel	ICTAHC	+++	++	+++	++
Italy	AIFA	++	+	+	+
South Korea	HIRA	++	+	+	+
Spain	CAHIRAQ (Catalan HTA Agency)	++	+	+	+
Sweden	TLV	++	+	++	+++
Taiwan	CDE	++	+	+++	++

Table 2. Overall assessment of HTA in selected markets

As RCTs are considered as gold standards, unpublished clinical trial data submitted in the dossier by the manufacturer is acceptable in many countries. However locally generated data from patient registries are increasing in importance, especially when the drug is entered to managed entry agreements.

9.3 Conclusions

In Table 2 is reported an overall assessment of HTA in selected markets. In all countries the main objective of Health Technology Assessment (HTA) is to conduct a systematic evaluation for a health technology in all aspects with a multidisciplinary approach in a transparent, unbiased manner to inform policy decisions. The role of HTA is also to provide input to market access decisions to determine reimbursement, funding level and price of a health technology, by informing payer bodies. In some cases, it's used as a determinant of the use of new technologies by providing guidance to prescribing specialists. HTA can ensure resources are used to fund the best medical technologies using the best clinical practice but one shouldn't overlook that all other stakeholders including, for example, physicians, pharmacists, patients and innovative pharmaceutical companies are impacted by the decisions.

4 References

1. International Working Group for HTA Advancement; Neumann PJ, Drummond MF, Jönsson B, et al. Are Key Principles for improved health technology assessment supported and used by health technology assessment organizations? *Int J Technol Assess Health Care* 2010; 26: 71-8
2. Nicod E, Kanavos P. Developing an evidence-based methodological framework to systematically compare HTA coverage decisions: A mixed methods study. *Health Policy* 2016; 120: 35-45
3. Hutton J, McGrath C, Frybourg JM, et al. Framework for describing and classifying decision-making systems using technology assessment to determine the reimbursement of health technologies (fourth hurdle systems). *Int J Technol Assess Health Care* 2006; 22: 10-8
4. European Federation of Pharmaceutical Industries and Associations (EFPIA). A comparative analysis of the role and impact of Health Technology Assessment (2011). Available at http://www.efpia.eu/uploads/Modules/Documents/hta-comparison-report-may-2011.pdf (last accessed September 2016)
5. Rutten F. Health technology assessment and policy from the economic perspective. *Int J Technol Assess Health Care* 2004; 20: 67-70
6. Velasco Garrido M, Gerhardus A, Røttingen JA, et al. Developing Health Technology Assessment to address health care system needs. *Health Policy* 2010; 94: 196-202
7. Haas M, Hall J, Viney R, et al. A model for best practice HTA. Working Papers 2008/1. Centre for Health Economics Research and Evaluation, University of Technology, Sydney. 2008

10. The Future of Market Access

Albert I. Wertheimer

Writing about the future is difficult. The writing itself is not difficult, but the accuracy part is difficult. On the other hand, even if the predictions are 100 percent wrong, it might not be until 5 or 10 years into the future when readers and others discover the inaccuracies. That reminds me of the ideal job: the television weather forecaster/reporter. It is the only job where one can be wrong more than 50 percent of the time and not lose one's job.

Hopefully, what we discuss in this chapter will come to pass. In any case, it is written with the author's best knowledge and judgment in 2016.

We will begin by discussing what is market access today and then we can explore what might be expected in the future. Market access is a term used to describe the various strategies and methods used by pharmaceutical companies to get access to purchasers of drugs, leaders who make formulary decisions and insurance and managed care personnel to enable their presentation or promotion of pharmaceutical products.

It is the same for companies in the diagnostics, devices, and biotechnology spaces. So, as a working definition, let us describe market access as the strategies and methods to enable communication with purchasers or deciders. It encompasses many routes that may or may not be used simultaneously depending on the individual circumstances.

10.1 The Market Access Avenues

Now, we consider market access made up by ten avenues, described in the future paragraphs:

1. Health Economics/Outcomes Research (HEOR).
2. Knowledgeable Opinion Leaders.
3. Value Pricing.
4. Value-added Services.
5. Joint Education/Prevention and Screening.
6. Personal Relationship Building.
7. Softening the Gatekeeper.
8. Advisory Board Membership.
9. Other/Assorted Strategies.
10. Pricing.

Health Economics

In the sphere of health economics, pharma companies today prepare dossiers and value proposition documents that attempt to demonstrate the superior virtues of their product compared with competing products. The rationale usually include one or more of the following attributes, among many others:

- Less costly than alternatives.
- Less costly array of adverse events.
- Enables shorter or eliminates hospitalization.
- Is not addictive.
- Minimally restrictive storage conditions.
- Simple or no preparation.
- Such as dosage calculation by weight.
- Better patient acceptance leading to better compliance.

In the future, this area is unlikely to change in any dramatic way in the next 5-10 years. There will be more precision as we move away from modeling and employ a greater reliance on Real-Word Data (RWD). RWD will be easier to obtain, cheaper to access and will be available sooner due to digital recording of clinical trial data and the new, more rigorous pharmacovigilance requirements for post-marketing experiences.

Perhaps the biggest change in health economics will be the separate calculations and reports for various gender and age group cohorts. Today, HEOR and Value Proposition reports are inclusive of all trail subjects or of the entire population who have used the drug since marketing approval. But, in the future, we will be able to generate reports on age groups divided by gender, such as males, 18-29 years, females 18-29 years, and by patient status such as those with hypertension in addition to their diabetes, those with heart failure, hypertension and diabetes for each age and gender cohort. That means that an insurer or Managed Care Organization (MCO) might select one drug for young adults, another for female seniors, etc.

Knowledgeable Opinion Leaders (KOLs)

This is a common strategy today to recruit KOLs to serve as advisors, members of speaker's bureau and as consultants. They are often included on HEOR publications even though they have had little or no role in the research or in the preparation of the research report manuscript. When a KOL speaks at a local medical society meeting and says positive things about a product, the thinking goes that if the speaker is respected by his or her peers, then other clinicians may try the drug with their own patients. Also it would be difficult for a KOL to laud the properties of one drug and prescribe a different drug in his or her practice.

Academic physicians are a prized category of KOLs. If they use a specific drug product, there is a high probability that their trainees/residents will become familiar with that same product and use it when they complete their formal training. Some people believe that if a well-regarded, local KOL is included as an author, that the publication of HEOR or clinical results will be more convincing than if all of the authors are unknown, from some distant country.

The future of this strategy is cloudy. Professional and scientific journals, more and more, are asking authors to certify that all listed authors actually contributed to the research or writing. The U.S. government now requires biopharmaceutical companies to list the amounts they pay to physicians each year and this information is then published in newspapers. Some physicians do not want to be seen as biopharmaceutical industry pawns. Moreover, the regulations are becoming so rigid that the company must prepare the slide deck and caution speakers about not deviating from the prepared script.

The use of KOLs will surely continue, but it is likely past its heyday. In addition, the charisma and reputation of a single practitioner is not sufficient to convince a health insurer or managed care organization to select one drug over another for formulary inclusion and reimbursement. That decision will be made based on dollars or euros.

Value Pricing

Value pricing is a newer market access tool which may have a very bright future. In simple terms, a pharmaceutical manufacturer will offer to cover the entire cost of care for a fixed number of hypertensive patients enrolled in a health insurance plan. Let us say that the cost of care for those hypertensive patients were $ 3.4 million last year. The offering company will say that they are so confident that their new product has superior effectiveness and a greater percentage of effectiveness, while also causing a lesser number of adverse events, that it offers to supply its drug to the MCO for $ 3.2 million. The manufacturer will keep a reserve cash fund to spend if the cost goes up, perhaps $ 200,000 and beyond that, the company buys reinsurance to spread the risk. If the total cost of care were to be $ 3.5 million, the MCO pays $ 3.2 million, the manufacturers pay $ 0.2 million and the insurer pays $ 100,000. However, next year the reinsurance firm premium will go up a great deal since the company had to pay out $ 100,000 in its initial year and expects history to repeat itself.

We can expect this value pricing methodology to increase, but instead of offers for all hypertensives in the plan, it is likely to consider the effect of personalized medicine on drug therapy. Therefore, the offer would be for treating all females 21-65 years of age, or for some other subpopulations of the society overall. This is also referred to as "risk sharing pricing". The manufacturer loves such joint arrangements as they typically permit the company and the clinicians to work more closely together in promoting the most cost-effective use of the drug, and in educating participating physicians for whom this drug should be used, where and when. Even if the pricing scheme was not profitable for the MCO, their physicians became familiar with the featured drug and may continue prescribing for MCO and non-MCO patients in the future.

Value-added Services

Many biopharmaceutical companies try to win favor and loyalty by giving gifts to insurers and managed care organizations. Most such gifts are non-cash. For example, they may assign company experts to assist with a computer system upgrade project; they may supply clinicians or researchers for Continuing Medical Education (CME) programs; they might provide reference books, print policy manuals, formularies, purchase a booth at a conference or symposium. This includes paying for consultants for the MCO, offering food or other refreshments at a staff meeting. Offering value-added services is quite commonplace today, and the value-added services can be in any realm; clinical, administrative, or educational, for example.

Value-added services' future is cloudy. Government agencies view some as illegal discounts which is illegal as it is price discrimination. In addition, in the U.S.A. and elsewhere, biopharmaceutical companies are required to give a specified price discount to government purchasers of drugs, with a requirement that no other commercial discounts can exceed that discount, and if they exceed it, the government purchaser must be given an equal discount. One could argue that a regular discount coupled with free, value-added services' value exceeds the maximum discount offered to government buyers. Recipients of value-added services are now expected to pay taxes on the estimated value of the services. Given, these, and other risks, from participating in offering value added services, it is reasonable to expect to witness a decline of value added service transactions. The concept will probably continue, but in all likelihood, it will be severely limited, constrained, and carefully evaluated.

Joint Education/Prevention and Screening

Pretend that XYZ Laboratories, a big seller of diabetes drugs, goes to a Health Maintenance Organization (HMO) or MCO to offer a joint educational program to potential diabetic patients. The program is open to the public, lay members of the health plan. The members learn the name of the company and undiagnosed patients now may become purchasers of the products if they are found to have elevated blood glucose levels. This is what is called a "win-win" situation. The plan gets good Public Relations (PR) for hosting a health evaluation festival day; the manufacturer gets new sales; and patients have free services to keep them healthy.

The manufacturer gets to work closely with KOLs and other clinicians and develops a good relationship with the plan officers.

Jointly sponsored programs such as learning to do productive exercise classes, smoking cessation, proper nutrition, stress reduction and more, help the health plan, the patients, and its physicians. These programs will likely grow and continue in the future. We see notices through our health insurers that will be an evening lecture on "you No Longer Need to Live With X Disease." Obviously, this program is sponsored by the makers of a new drug intended for treatment of that condition. Just as seen in this example, the marketer is attempting a "pull" strategy. The usual "push" promotional strategy is aimed at reaching prescribers and insurance company deciders. This "pull" strategy aims at patients/consumer to ask their physicians to prescribe a drug for them that they saw advertised on television. Direct-to Consumer advertising is effective and grows larger each year. As a rule, physicians dislike it since the requested drug may not be needed by the patient, and insurers like it less, as the practice increases their medication cost per patient.

Personal Relationship Building

The creation of personal relationships is probably one of the most successful and powerful tools available to the biopharmaceutical company. The company representative learns that the physician is a huge football fan. The representative will insert football into the conversation to augment a rapport between them and no one should be surprised to learn that the company has given two football game tickets as a holiday or birthday present. Sales representatives are frequently selected for their wholesome looks, good sense of humor, and interaction skills. After the football tickets, the representative feels free to say to the physician that his/her company is holding a competition this month and the representative would be grateful if the physicians could prescribe more of Drug A to appropriate patients, if possible for this month.

This will increase in the future. While a field force is costly, it has been proven to be effective in generating sales of the companies' products. Logically, a representative may only see 4-6 prescribers per day. The company pays a salary, an automobile, fringe benefits, training expense, samples and other literature, as well as travel to periodic meetings. This large cost must generate sales and profits in excess of the cost, or it would have been abandoned years ago. The message may be controlled more in the future by using a laptop computer to deliver a standard message that is vetted by the legal department for regulatory compliance and clinical accuracy and fairness/balance.

Softening the Gatekeeper

Most physician practices and clinics have a practice manager who supervises the day-to-day functioning of the office, managing the staff, handling financial matters and serving as a gatekeeper to the actual physicians. To get face-to-face time with the physician depends often on the attitude of that gatekeeper toward the representative. Those liked by the practice manager get to chat with the physician with minimal waiting and sometimes for a longer meeting duration. Others may face hours and hours of unproductive time in a waiting room chair, or be told to return on another day.

The gatekeeper's opinion of the representative is formed by the representative proving that they respect the practice manager and her important role. It is added to by the representative bringing small, thoughtful gifts such as a box lunch or pizza for the staff in the office, OTC cold and cough medicines for their children or family. Successful representatives work with the practice manager and do not try to out-maneuver or circumvent their authority. The smart representative brings samples when learning that Uncle George has a dermatitis, or buying tickets when someone's kids are selling lottery tickets for a school fund raising campaign. The chance of the representative hearing: "The doctor can see you now. He had a cancellation and you can have up to 10 minutes right now" is enhanced by good relations with the office staff.

Advisory Boards

In the recent past, physicians have been invited to lovely settings; golf courses, beach resorts, historical cities, cruises and similar venues where they served as an advisory board member, ostensibly to provide their feedback and opinions about a new product. Most observers viewed this as a strategy to gather a captive audience and use the face time to promote a product or products, while providing an opportunity for the physician to enjoy a destination vacation for a weekend. However, recently, the US Food and Drug Administration (FDA) has cracked down on this activity. Spouses have to travel and stay/dine at their own expense, and then non-presenters could not receive company funding. Since these are very expensive endeavors and only a small number of physicians participate each time, it is losing favor and nearly all biopharmaceutical companies have reduced the number of advisory board meetings.

In the future, expect advisory board meetings to become rare. They will be held to teach physicians how to use new technologies, diagnostic devices or entirely new classes of drugs or new dosage forms, such as inhaled insulins, therapeutic vaccines, robotic procedures, new Intra-Uterine Device insertion, etc. They may continue in a different format on line via Skype or Go-to-Meeting, which are clearly far cheaper and more efficient.

Other Market Access Endeavors

Pharma companies will make donations to a physician's favorite charity, offer customized courses of study to MCO clinicians and administrators, to be held at the premises of the health plan, at a time convenient to the audience. In this day of inflation and rapidly increasing prices of drug products, some companies will offer price guarantees for a specified period of time, commonly 1-2 years. So even if the price increases across the board, that health insurer will continue to be able to buy the drug at the current agreed-upon price, or else a rebate will be provided by the manufacturer so that the expenditure remains the same.

Related to this practice is the strategy of volume based discounts or rebates. If the MCO generates 50% market share, it receives 10 cents per tablet back as a reward discount. It might be 15 cents for a 70% market share, and 25 cents if the plan reaches a 90% market level and places that drug in its preferred formulary position with the smallest patient co-payment level.

While this has been profitable for companies in the past, it has now become a massive expense to them in rebate costs as well as supporting a large department to negotiate and administer the agreements. Most industry observers believe that the firms would pounce on an opportunity to change their rebate obligations to a new metric at lower cost.

Several US States have enacted legislation requiring Pharmacy Benefit Managers (PBMs), the pharmacy sector agency of Managed Care Organizations, to provide transparency and report the sources of their income. Such visibility decreases the incentive for manufacturers to enter into private rebate agreements, unknown to the public or to their competitors.

Pricing

Perhaps the oldest and simplest strategy is that of offering the lowest price for a drug product. Until now, this was possible only with generic drugs, since they are considered to be equivalent and interchangeable. 50 mg tablets of losartan, if government agency approved should be bioequivalent to any other losartan 50 mg tablets, enabling the health insurer to purchase the lowest priced option from among the multiple suppliers of the standardized, commodity product.

This has not been possible with branded new products until recently. When there is more than one product for an indication, large health insurers are beginning to pit them against each other and will pay for the one agent at the lowest net price to them. This came to light in early 2015, when a drug used to cure hepatitis C went on the market for $ 84,000 for a 12-week course of therapy. Shortly thereafter two other manufacturers were authorized to see their similar, but not identical hepatitis C products. The PBMs negotiated strongly and ended up placing only one of those drugs on its formulary. It is estimated that they pay at least $ 20,000 less for this exclusive position. Large purchasers can be expected to do this with new, costly therapeutic vaccines, and oncology drugs.

0.2 Conclusion

There are numerous other market access strategies evolving or declining. While they differ, often in multiple ways, they generally fit into one of the categories covered earlier in this chapter. For the next three-to-five years, we should not expect any radical changes in the current market access tools as they would be known today and more than likely, they would be pilot tested this year or soon. We see more evolution than revolution in business, especially in the healthcare space.

Just as the doctor house call has nearly disappeared because of the "wasted" travel time between patients, in-person detail person visits may become virtual as well. The house call doctor might see 6-8 patients per day, while a physician in his/her office can see six per hour or at least 40 in a single day. And lastly, as the nature of therapeutics evolves, we may witness more specialized physician types who only deal in regenerative medicine, genetic therapies, therapeutic vaccines, requiring a much smaller population of very highly trained company representatives in these ultra-specialized areas in the future.

0.3 To know more

- Academy of Managed Care Pharmacy. www.amcp.org (last accessed October 2015)
- American Cancer Society. www.americancancersociety.org (last accessed October 2015)

- Biotechnology Industry Organization. www.BIO.org (last accessed October 2015)
- Fulda TR, Wertheimer A. Handbook of Pharmaceutical Public Policy. Cleveland, OH: CRC Press, Taylor and Francis Group, 2007
- Kongstvedt PR. Health Insurance and Managed Care: What they are and How they Work. Burlington, MA: Jones and Bartlett, 2015, 4th Edition
- Luft HS. Health Maintenance Organizations: Dimensions of Performance. New Brunswick, NJ: Transaction Books, 1987
- Navarro RP. Managed Care Pharmacy Practice. Boston, MA: Jones & Bartlett, 2009, 2nd Edition
- Pharmaceutical Research and Manufacturers of America®. www.PhRMA.org (last accessed October 2015)
- Pradelli L, Wertheimer A. Pharmacoeconomics: Principles and Practice. Torino, Italy: SEEd Medical Publishers, 2012
- Rychlik R. Strategies in Pharmacoeconomics and Outcomes Research. Cleveland, OH: CRC Press, Taylor and Francis Group, 2002
- Smith MI, Wertheimer A, Fincham JE. Pharmacy and the US Health Care System. London, England: Pharmaceutical Press, 2013, 4th Edition
- Vogel RJU. Pharmaceutical Economics and Public Policy. New York (NY): Haworth Press, 2007
- Wertheimer A, Navarro RP. Managed Care Pharmacy: Principles and Practice. Cleveland, OH: CRC Press, Taylor and Francis Group, 1999

11. Conclusions

Güvenç Koçkaya
With the collaboration of Kagan Atikeler

The definition of market access was reported by the World Trade Organization as "to open markets for trade and improve transparency, reciprocity and non-discrimination in international trade" [1]. Nowadays, market access has a critical role for pharmaceutical companies. If decision makers which are mostly public payers will not allow the reimbursement of a product to a broader population or at an optimum price for the company, marketing and sales activities cannot be effective.

The market access process in Emerging Countries was tried to be defined in this book with 6 different chapters while there were some limitations. The first limitation is that it is not possible to include all emerging countries in one book. However, the book included 26 emerging countries which are the most important markets in their regions. The second limitation is the book was not reviewed by government authorities from each country. However, authors are experts on their topics.

Multinational pharmaceutical companies launch new products in emerging countries mostly after developed world launches. The time difference was reported as 1.25 years [2]. This time difference may have a negative effect as patents expire in emerging markets with launching of generics. However, it was reported that multinational companies have opportunity with branded generics in emerging countries [2]. It was reported in another report that while original molecules have a compound annual growth rate (CAGR) as 8.6%, the generics had 15% in emerging countries between 2010-2012 [3].

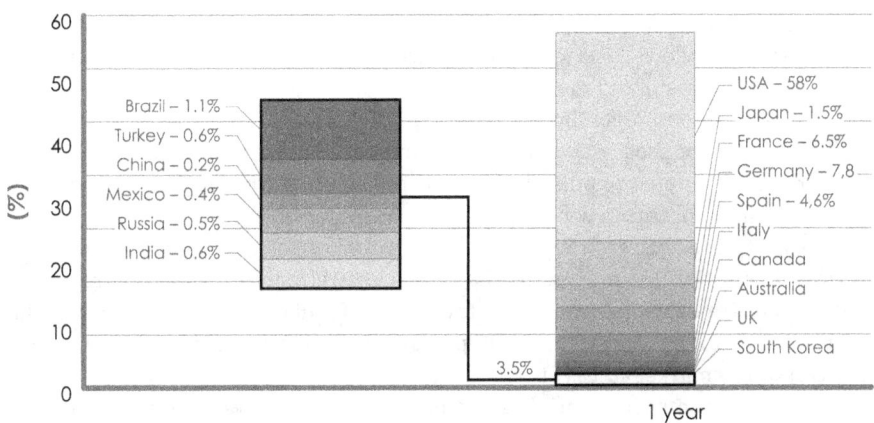

Figure 1. Pharmaceutical Sales Depending on IMS Health Report [4]

It is clear that emerging countries are important for the multinational pharmaceutical companies. It was reported that CAGR of 6.0 per cent in the period from 2011-2017, and expected sales exceeding USD 1.1 trillion by 2017 [4]. Brazil, Turkey, China, Mexico, Russia and India are 3,5% of global first year sales of original products (Figure 1) [4]. In addition, CAGR 2008-2012 for recent launched pharmaceuticals were 9,8% and 1.5% in Emerging Countries and top 8 developed countries (US, Japan, France, Germany, Spain, Italy, Canada, Australia), respectively [3].

Emerging countries can`t be ignored by multinational pharmaceutical companies for launching new products. So the market access process in these countries will be important in near future also.

Market access is a bit different issue for least developed countries. The biggest barriers to access and improved health are not drug prices or patents but "on the ground" barriers such as market failure, corruption, non-existent health human resources and infrastructure, and the lack of both local and international political will [4]. The most significant improvements have been seen on public-private partnerships (PPPs). The PPPs are helping to improve access to medicines in the least developed countries [4]. Low income countries gain a lot for both access to medicines and health outcomes with various PPPs [4]. It has been reported that there are 150 PPPs to improve access to medicine in least developed countries and most of them industry-led agreements [4]. Doha Declaration which made compulsory licensing unnecessary resulted with incentive of PPPs since 2003 [4].

Some countries such as Indonesia, Brazil and Argentina produce their own generics in government owned factories in order to prevent public health problems and create environment for patient access to innovative medicines [5]. Given the benefits of the 'government use' provisions for access to drugs, the government together with health groups should pursue similar measures for essential drugs in Indonesia [5].

It was reported in a pharmaceutical industry survey in which top 15 pharmaceutical companies holding 50% of market shares participated [6]. Lack of reimbursement of public funding and infrastructure are reported as the main concerns of pharmaceutical market access in emerging markets.[6] 68% of the participants responded as lack of funding is main problem that followed by lack of infrastructure by 67% [6]. Making local investment as research, development and manufacturing is seen as a tool for effective market access success in these regions depending of 60% of participants [6]. The lack of transparency, unpredicted length of processes of tendering and contracting are reported as other factors also [6,7]. It is offered to publish all government contracts regarding the use of public property and finances to reverse the lack of transparency [8].

It was easy to see that each region and each country has specific environments and conditions. Market access process in the countries are mostly defined by regulations. However, there are examples not fitting the written regulations like delaying timelines, additional discounts, etc. For that, it is important to understand the culture of a country to be successful in market access also.

One of the most important hurdles in emerging countries was reported as Pricing & Market Access in many reports. This situation may maintain in near future also [3,5,6]. Depending on the needs, it is possible to make a global market access strategy for the pharmaceutical countries from headquarters but not possible to implement the global strategies without local tactics. For implementing local tactics, it is needed to involve local experts in each region or each countries. This book may help the local experts who are beginning or in middle of their careers, the government officers who are looking at new implementations, and the headquarters managements who want to learn more about emerging markets.

1.1 **References**

1. World Trade Organization. Available at http://www.wto.org (Last accessed August 2015)
2. Chemtech Foundation. Strategies for Successful Launch of New Pharmaceutical Products in Emerging Markets. Available at http://www.chemtech-online.com/P&B/Manish_april13.html (Last accessed August 2015)
3. IMS Health. Pharmerging markets. Picking a pathway to success. Available at https://www.imshealth.com/files/web/Global/Services/Services%20TL/IMS_Pharmerging_WP.pdf (Last accessed August 2015)
4. Taylor W. Pharmaceutical Access in Least Developed Countries: on-the-ground barriers and industry successes. The Cameron Institute, 2010. Available at http://apps.who.int/medicinedocs/documents/s17815en/s17815en.pdf (Last accessed August 2015)
5. Hanim L, Jhamtani H. Indonesia: Manufacturing generic AIDS medicines under the 'Government Use' approach. Third World Resurgence, 2006. Available at http://www.citizen.org/documents/CL%20in%20Indonesia%202004.pdf (Last accessed August 2015)
6. Buente M, Danner S, Weissbäcker S, et al. Pharma emerging markets 2.0, How emerging markets are driving the transformation of the pharmaceutical industry. Booz & Company, 2013. Available at http://www.strategyand.pwc.com/media/file/Strategyand_Pharma-Emerging-Markets-2.0.pdf (Last accessed August 2015)
7. Mujal A. Pharma Faces Hurdles in Emerging Markets. Synapse, 2016. Available at http://synapse.ucsf.edu/articles/2016/01/04/pharma-faces-hurdles-emerging-markets (Last accessed August 2015)
8. Center for Global Development (CGDev). Publishing Government Contracts. Addressing Concerns and Easing Implementation. A Report of the Center for Global Development. CGDev, 2014. Available at http://www.cgdev.org/publication/ft/publishing-government-contracts-addressing-concerns-and-easing-implementation (Last accessed August 2015)

Glossary

ABF	Activity-Based Funding
ACE	Angiotensin-Converting-Enzyme
AHTAPol	National Agency for Health Technology Assessment and Tarification (Poland)
AIFD	*Araştırmacı İlaç Firmaları Derneği'nin* (Association of Research-Based Pharmaceutical Companies)
AMRP	Abbreviated Medicine Review Process (South Africa)
AMU	Arab Maghreb Union
ANAMED	Agencia nacional de medicamentos (Chile)
ANMAT	Administración Nacional de Medicamentos, Alimentos y Tecnología Médica (Argentina)
ANVISA	Agência Nacional de Vigilância Sanitária (Brazil)
APL	Approved Product List (South Africa)
ARRA	American Recovery and Reinvestment Act
ATP	Market-based Actual Transaction Pricing (South Korea)
BHFPC	Bureau Health and Family Planning Commission (China)
BHRSS	Bureau Human Resources and Social Security (China)
BMI	Body Mass Index
BRIC	Brazil, Russia, India, and China
CA	Commercial Agreements
CAGR	Compounded Average Growth Rate
CAPA	Central Administration for Pharmaceutical Affairs (Egypt)
CCS	Cooperative of Civil Servants (Lebanon).
CDE	Centre for Drug Evaluation (China)
CED	Coverage with Evidence Development
CFDA	China Food and Drug Administration (China)
cGMP	current Good Manufacturing Practice
CHC	Community Health Centers (China)
CHIP	Children's Health Insurance Program
CIF	Cost, Insurance and Freight (UAE)
CIP	Civil health Insurance Program (Jordan)
CME	Continuing Medical Education
CMKP	*Centrum Medyczne Kształcenia Podyplomowego* (Medical Centre of Postgraduate Education)
CMS	Centres for Medicare & Medicaid Services (U.S.A.)
CMS	Council for Medical Schemes (South Africa)
COFEPRIS	Comisión Federal para la Protección contra Riesgos Sanitarios (Mexico)
CONITEC	Comissão Nacional de Incorporação de Tecnologias

CPP	Certificate of Pharmaceutical Product
CPU	Clinical Policy Unit (South Africa)
CSIOZ	Center for Health Information Systems
CSLL	Contribuição Social sobre o Lucro Líquido (Brazil)
CSMBS	Civil Servants Medical Benefits Scheme (Thailand)
CTD	Common Technical Dossier
DAA	Directly Acting Antiviral
DALY	Disability-Adjusted Life Year
DHA	Dubai Health Authority (UAE)
DIGEMID	Dirección General de Medicamentos, Insumos y Drogas (Perù)
DM	Diabetes Mellitus
DMS	voluntary medical insurance (Russia)
DoH	Department of Health
DRG	Diagnosis-Related Group
DUR	Drug Utilization Review (South Korea)
EAC	East African Community
EAN	International Article Number
ECOWAS	Economic Community Of West African States
EDA	Egyptian Drug Authority (Egypt)
EDL	Essential Drug List
EMA	European Medicines Agency (UE)
EMA	European Medicines Agency (UE)
EMCI	Essential Medical Cost Index (Thailand)
EMIT	Emergency Medical Institute of Thailand (Thailand)
EML	Essential Medicines List (South Africa)
EMP	Equal Maximum Price (South Korea)
EMP	Essential Medicines Programme (South Africa)
EMU	Economic and Monetary Union
EPR	External Price Referencing
EPS	Entidades Promotoras de Salud (Colombia)
ERP	External Reference Pricing
ES	*Emekli Sandığı* (Pension Fund – Turkey)
ES	Equitable Share (South Africa)
FAP	*Feldshersko-Akusherskiy Punkt* (feldsher-midwife posts)
FCCCER	Federal Coordinating Council for Comparative Effectiveness Research
FDA	Food and Drug Administration (USA)
FFOMS	Federal Fund for Mandatory Medical Insurance
FMBA	Federal Medical and Biological Agency
FOSYGA	Fondo de Seguridad y Garantía en Salud (Colombia)
GCC	Gulf Cooperation Council
GCC-GP	GCC Group Purchasing (GCC)
GDP	Gross Domestic Product
GIS	Government Insurance Scheme (China)

GLP	Good Laboratory Practice
GMP	Good Manufacturing Practice
GPMM	Government Price Method for Medicines (China)
GPO	Government Pharmaceutical Organization (Thailand)
HAAD	Health Authority Abu Dhabi (UAE)
HCS	HealthCare System (UAE)
HCV	Hepatitis C Virus
HEOR	Health Economics/Outcomes Research
HIO	Health Insurance Organization (Egypt)
HIRA	Health Insurance Review & Assessment Service (South Korea)
HIS	Health Information System (UAE)
HITAP	Health Intervention and Technology Assessment Program (Thailand)
HMC	Health Ministers' Council (GCC)
HMO	Health Maintenance Organization
HSRO	Health System Research Institute (Thailand)
HT	Health Technology
HTA	Health Technology Assessment
HTP	Health Transformation Program
ICER	Incremental Cost-Effectiveness Ratio
ICH	International Council on Harmonisation of technical requirements for registration of pharmaceuticals for human use
IETS	Instituto de Evaluación Tecnológica en Salud
IFC	International Financial Corporation
IMSS	Instituto Mexicano del Seguro Social (Mexico)
INN	International Non-proprietary Name
INVIMA	Instituto Nacional de Vigilancia de Medicamentos y Alimentos (Colombia)
IPASME	Instituto de Prevensión y Asistencia Social del Ministerio de Educación, Cultura y Deportes (Venezuela)
IPSFA	Instituto de Prevención Social de las Fuerzas Armadas (Venezuela)
ISafE	Information, SAFety and ease of use, Efficacy (Thailand)
iSEM	in-hospital Surgical and Ethical Management (South Africa)
ISP	Chile's Instituto de Salud Pública
ISPOR	International Society of Pharmacoeconomics and Outcomes Research
ISSSTE	Instituto de Seguridad y Servicios Sociales de los Trabajadores del Estado (Mexico)
İTS	*İlaç Takip Sistemi* (Pharmaceuticals Electronic Tracking System) (Turkey)
IVSS	Instituto Venezolano de los Seguros Sociales
JCI	Joint Commission International
JFDA	Jordanian Food and Drug Administration (Jordan)
KFDA	Korea Food and Drug Administration (South Korea)
KOL	Key Opinion Leader
KPI	Key Performance Indicator

KSA	Kingdom of Saudi Arabia
LIS	Labor Insurance Scheme (China)
MAA	Market Access Agreements
MAH	Market Authorization Holder (UAE)
MATP	Market-based Actual Transaction Pricing (South Korea)
MCC	Medicines Control Council (South Africa)
MCO	Managed Care Organization
ME	Middle East
MENA	Middle East and North Africa region
MFDS	Ministry of Food and Drug Safety (South Korea)
MHI	Mandatory Health Insurance
MHLW	Ministry of Health, Labor and Welfare (Japan)
MID	Mandatory Institutional Discount
MIT	Ministry of Industry and Trade
MoF	Ministry of Finance
MoH	Ministry of Health
MOHP	Ministry of Health and Population (Egypt)
MOHRSS	Ministry of Human Resources and Social Security (China)
MoHSD	Ministry of Health and Social Development
MOHWFA	Ministry Of Health, Welfare and Family Affairs (South Korea)
MOL&SS	Ministry of Labor and Social Security
MoPH	Ministry of Public Health
MPR	Medicine Price Registry (South Africa)
MS	Multiple Sclerosis
MSAC	Medical Services Advisory Commission (Australia)
NAFDAC	National Agency for Food and Drug Administration and Control (Nigeria)
NAFTA	North American Free Trade Agreement
NAPAMS	Nigerian Automated Product And Monitoring Solutions (Nigeria)
NAPPI	National Pharmaceutical Product Index (South Africa)
NCD	Non-Communicable Disease
NCE	New Chemical Entity (South Africa)
NDC	National Diabetes Centre (KSA)
NDRC	National Development and Reform Commission (China)
NDSDC	National Drug System Development Committee (Thailand)
NECA	National Evidence based healthcare Collaborating Agency (South Korea)
NEDL	National Essential Drug List (China)
NEMLC	National Essential Medicines List Committee (South Africa)
NFZ	National Health Fund (Poland)
NGO	non-governmental organization
NGO	Non-Governmental Organization
NHCO	National Health Commission Office (Thailand)
NHFPC	National Health and Family Planning Commission (China)

NHI	National Health Insurance
NHIC	National Health Insurance Corporations (South Korea)
NHLS	National Health Laboratory Service (South Africa)
NHSO	National Health Security Office (Thailand)
NIZP	National Institute of Public Health
NLED	National List of Essential Drugs (Thailand)
NODCAR	National Organization for Drug Control and Research (Egypt)
NORCB	National Organization for Research and Control of Biologicals (Egypt)
NPFPC	National Population and Family Planning Commission (China)
NPP	National Priority Project (Russia)
NRA	National Regulatory Authority
NRCMS	New Rural Cooperative Medical Scheme (China)
NRDL	National Reimbursement Drug List (China)
NRS	National Regulatory Systems
NSSF	National Social Security Fund (Lebanon)
OECD	Organization for Economic Cooperation and Development
OFT	Office of Fair Trading
OMS	mandatory medical insurance (Russia)
OOP	Out-Of-Pocket
OPS	Organización Panamericana de la Salud
OPSDC	Office of the Public Sector Development Commission (Thailand)
OTC	Over The Counter
P&R	pricing and reimbursement
P4P	Payment for Performance
PAHO	Pan American Health Organization
PAMI-INSSJP	Programa de Atención Médica Integral-Instituto Nacional de Servicios Sociales para Jubilados y Pensionados (Argentina)
PAS	Patient Access Scheme
PBM	Pharmacy Benefit Manager
PCT	Primary Care Trust
PE	pharmacoeconomic
PEDL	Provincial Essential Drug List (China)
PHD	Provincial Health Department (South Africa)
PhRMA	Pharmaceutical Research and Manufacturers of America
PIN	Product Introduction Notification (South Africa)
PMB	Prescribed Minimum Benefit (South Africa)
PMDA	Pharmaceuticals and Medical Devices Agency
PMO	Programa Médico Obligatorio (Argentina)
POS	Plan Obligatorio de Salud (Colombia)
PPP	Public-Private Partnership
PR	Public Relations
PRDL	Provincial Reimbursement Drug List (China)
PROFE	PROgrama FEderal de Salud (Argentina)

PTC	Pharmacy and Therapeutics Committee (South Africa)
PVA	Price-Volume Agreement (South Korea)
PZH	National Institute of Hygiene
QALY	Quality Adjusted Life Years
QCL	Quality Control Laboratory
RBRV	Resource-Based Relative Value (South Korea)
RC	Reference Ceiling
REC	Regional Economic Community
Red-PARF	Red Pan Americana de Armonización Farmacéutica
RMS	Royal Medical Services (Jordan)
RSDE	Rewards for Saving Drug Expenditure (South Korea)
RWD	Real-Word Data
SADC	South African Development Community (South Africa)
SAHPRA	South African Health Products Regulatory Authority (South Africa)
SAUMP	State Administration of Ukraine on Medicinal Products (Ukraine)
SBRA	Summary Basis for Regulatory Action (South Africa)
SEHA	Abu Dhabi Health Services (UAE)
SEP	Single Exit Price (South Africa)
SFDA	State Food and Drug Administration (China)
SFDA	Saudi Food and Drug Authority (KSA)
SGH	Secretariat General Health (Gulf Cooperation Council)
SGK	*Sosyal Güvenlik Kurumu* (Social Security Institution) (Turkey)
SHI	Social Health Insurance (South Korea)
SPNS	Sistema Público Nacional de Salud (Venezuela)
SSA	Sub-Saharan Africa
SSI	Social Security Institution (*Sosyal Güvenlik Kurumu*)
SSK	*Sosyal Sigortalar Kurumu* (Social Insurance Institution)
SSO	Social Security Office (Thailand)
SSS	Social Security Scheme (Thailand)
STGs	Standard Treatment Guidelines (South Africa)
SUS	Sistema Único de Sâude (Brazil)
T2DM	ype 2 Diabetes Mellitus
TB	Tuberculosis
TGA	Therapeutic Goods Administration (Australia)
THE	Total Healthcare Expenditure
TİTCK	*Türkiye İlaç ve Tıbbi Cihaz Kurumu* (Turkish Pharmaceuticals and Medical Devices Agency)
TKHK	*Türkiye Kamu Hastaneleri Kurumu* (Turkish Public Hospitals Authority)
TPHA	urkısh Public Hospitals Authority (*Türkiye Kamu Hastaneleri Kurumu*)
TPMDA	Turkısh Pharmaceuticals and Medical Devices Agency (*Türkiye İlaç ve Tıbbi Cihaz Kurumu*)
TRT	Thai Rak Thai (Thailand)
UAE	United Arab Emirates

UBHIS	Urban Basic Health Insurance Scheme (China)
UCS	Universal Coverage Scheme (Thailand)
UEBMI	Urban Employee Basic Medical Insurance (China)
UMC	Uppsala Monitoring Center
UNASUR	Union of South American Nations
UNRWA	United Nation Relief and Works Agency
UPFS	Uniform Patient Fee Schedule (South Africa)
URAC	Utilization Review Accreditation Commission (UAE)
URBMI	Urban Residents Basic Medical Insurance (China)
URPLWMiPB	The Office for Registration of Pharmaceuticals, Medical Devices and Biocidal Products (Poland)
VAT	Value-Added Tax
VIP	Value Incentive Program (South Korea)
VOC	Verification Of Conformity (Kenya)
WAP	Weighted Average Price (South Korea)
WDF	World Diabetes Foundation
WHO	World Health Organization
WSP	WholeSale Price
WTO	World Trade Organization
YLD	Years Lost due to Disability
YLL	Years of Life Lost
YMCA	Young Men's Christian Association

Authors

Ola Al Ahdab

Dr Ola Al Ahdab is UAE national working as a Pharmaceutical Advisor at drug department, Ministry of Health, Abu Dhabi, United Arab Emirates. She has held several positions across the MOH since 199. Dr. Al Ahdab work as adjunct assistant professor of pharmacy practice in three universities (Sharjah, Ajman and Dubai Pharmacy College) in the UAE. Dr. Al Ahdab Post graduate studies were completed at Queens University of Belfast, UK, School of Pharmacy, where she was awarded a PhD in Pharmacoeconomics and Medicine Management in December 2008 as a full time study, and Post Graduate Diploma in Clinical Pharmacy in December 2003 as part time study. Furthermore, she has been awarded an honorary Postdoctoral Research Fellow at Clinical and Practice Research Centre, School of Pharmacy, Queens University of Belfast, United Kingdom. She has completed her undergraduate studies from the Damascus University, School of Pharmacy. Dr. Ola is an active member in many international professional organizations such as the International Society of Pharmacoeconomics and Outcomes Research (ISPOR). She is the founding president of the UAE ISPOR chapter established in April 2011, the International Pharmaceutical Federation (FIP), in addition, she is the Vice-President for Pharmacy Society, Emirates Medical Association UAE

Taric Catic

Tarik Čatić is a young researcher and consultant in the field of health economics, pharmacoeconomics, HTA, and market access. His area of expertise include marketing, sales and market access in the field of oncology, rheumatoid arthritis, neurology and rare diseases. His specific areas of interests are market access of innovative medicines, risk sharing schemes, modeling and outcomes research as well as health policy. He has participated as invited lecturers in numerous congresses and conferences and published more than 20 papers in scientific journals. He has established ISPOR Bosnia and Herzegovina Chapter and he has been the first president (2011-2015) of it. He has participated in the translation of ISPOR books into Bosnian, ISPOR distance learning programs, and Good Practices documents. He organized pharmacoeconomics conferences and courses and participated in some educational and researching projects.

Güvenç Koçkaya

Dr Güvenç Koçkaya is a medical doctor and health economist. He earned a master of science degree in Pharmacoeconomics & Pharmacoepidemiology at Yeditepe University and doctorate degree in Clinical Pharmacology and Medical Pharmacology at Istanbul University. He completed the European Market Access Diploma Program at Lyon-1 University and studied as a short term fellow at Temple University's Center for Pharmaceutical Health Services Research. He has established the ISPOR Yeditepe University Student Section. In 2011, he became the first Turkish citizen to be awarded the "ISPOR Meeting Travel Scholarship Award." He has several articles and posters that have been published in national and international journals or presented in national and international congresses. He has also served as the Turkish translation editor of Bootman`s Principles of Pharmacoeconomics and WHO`s Health Technology Assessment in Medical Devices. He worked for Ministry of Health of Turkey as health economist and a member of Medical and Economic Evaluation Commission, which evaluates pharmaceutical reimbursement decisions. He worked also as head of market access or health economics department in pharmaceutical & medical device companies. He is the President of the Health Economics and Policy Association (HEPA) and plays an active role in the development of health economics in Turkey and a member of scientific advisory board of "Farmeconomia. Health economics and therapeutic pathways".

Debra Leong

Debra Leong is a Market Planning Manager at the Market Analysis & Strategy group at Genentech. She graduated with both a M.S. and B.S. degree in Biomedical Engineering from Columbia University, with a focus on cell and tissue engineering. Prior to joining Genentech, Debra was a Managing Consultant in the Life Sciences practice of Navigant Consulting (formerly Easton Associates), where she specialized in market access and reimbursement strategy with expertise across APAC, LatAm, EU and EMEA, including South Africa. Debra has presented at several international conferences on market access strategy and also co-authored an article on market access for medical devices.

Mete Saylan

Mete Saylan had his medical doctor degree in Istanbul University Medical Faculty and he finished his specialization in psychiatry at Istanbul Medical Faculty Psychiatry Department. He started his academic career with clinical research in neurosciences. In 2001, he joined pharmaceutical industry as clinical research physician and he worked in medical and market access department of different international pharmaceutical companies. He's currently Market Access Director of Turkey, Iran and Maghreb countries.

Arturo Schweiger

Arturo Schweiger is a Health Economist that holds a MA degree in Economic Policy at Boston University with a Fulbright Scholarship. He has worked for the Interamerican Development Bank (IDB) and the Pan-American Health Organization (PAHO) in South American countries. Nowadays holds a position as senior auditor on social programs financed by Multilateral Organizations at the Auditoria General de la Nación (AGN), BS. As. Argentina. He is the director of the master course in Health Economics Management at Universidad Isalud – Bs. As. Argentina, and author of publication, thesis director and research projects. He has been president of the Argentina Health Economic Association (2004-2006) and foundational member of the Board the Health Economics Association (2008)"

Mondher Toumi

Professor Mondher Toumi is M.D. by training, M.Sc. in Biostatistics, and in Biological Sciences (option pharmacology) and Ph.D. in Economic Sciences. Mondher Toumi is Professor of Public Health at Aix-Marseille University.

After working for 12 years as Research Manager in the department of pharmacology at the University of Marseille, he joined the Public Health Department in 1993. In 1995 he embraces a carrier in the pharmaceutical industry for 13 years. Mondher Toumi was appointed Global Vice President at Lundbeck A/S in charge of health economics, outcome research, pricing, market access, epidemiology, risk management, governmental affairs and competitive intelligence. In 2008, he founded Creativ-Ceutical, an international consulting firm dedicated to support health industries and authorities in strategic decision-making. In February 2009 he was appointed Professor at Lyon I University in the Department of Decision Sciences and Health Policies. The same year, he was appointed Director of the Chair of Public Health and Market Access. He launched the first European University Diploma of Market Access (EMAUD) an international course already followed by almost 350 students. Additionally, he recently created the Market Access Society to promote education, research and scientific activities at the interface of market access, HTA, public health and health economic assessment. He is editor in Chief of the Journal of Market Access and Health Policy (JMAHP) which was just granted PubMed indexation. Mondher Toumi is also visiting Professor at Beijing University (Third Hospital). He is a recognized expert in health economics and an authority on market access and risk management. He authored more than 250 scientific publications and communications, and has contributed to several books.

Esin Tuna

Esin Tuna is currently working as a consultant in Polar Health Economics and Policy Consultancy Company based in Ankara from December 2013. Polar is a consultancy company providing research, consultancy, and training services in all social policy issues with special reference to health care. Main areas of work include consultancy and training in health technology assessment, health economics and pharmacoeconomic analyses, reimbursement/market access, pricing, policy analysis, health care financing and costing studies and market research. Prior to Polar, she worked at Bayer Pharma as a Health Policy Specialist between 2012 and 2013. She received her BSc degree from Hacettepe University Faculty of Pharmacy in 2011. She has master degrees on "Health Economics and Pharmacoeconomics" and "Biopharmaceutics and Pharmacokinetics". She has national and international publications on health economics and policy issues.

Albert Wertheimer

Professor Albert Wertheimer is a professor at the College of Pharmacy, Nova Southeastern University, Lauderdale, FL, USA. His area of expertise include pharmacoeconomics, outcome research, managed care pharmacy, pharmaceutical health services research, and international health policy. He had served as Professor at the Temple University and at the University of Minnesota, Dean at the Philadelphia College of Pharmacy, Director of Health Outcomes Management at Merck and Company, Director of the Center for Pharmaceutical Health Services Research, and vice president of Pharmacy Managed Care First Health. He received a Bachelor of Pharmacy degree from the University of Buffalo; a Master of Business Administration from the State University of New York at Buffalo, and a PhD degree from Purdue University. He was also a post-doctoral fellow at the Department of Social Medicine at St. Thomas' Hospital Medical School of the University of London (UK). He is author of 29 books, more than 420 article in scientific journals, and more than 30 book chapters. He has supervised 70 PhD Students and 104 Master degree students. Professor Wertheimer has consulted or lectured in over 60 countries.

Kally Wong

Kally Wong entered consumer and media research early in the career. Specialized in market analysis for the pharmaceutical industry about 15 years ago. She has worked in 7 countries span across the Asia Pacific and European region. Kally is now based in Basel, Switzerland.

Fatma Betul Yenilmez

Fatma Betul Yenilmez studied nursing at Koc University, Turkey. Her job experiences comprise nursing and sales&marketing in pharmaceuticals. Her educational background also includes master degrees and lots of certificates in both nursing and health economics. She has worked as a consultant both for government and private sector since 2014. She published several scientific posters and articles in health economics and market access area.

www.ingramcontent.com/pod-product-compliance
Lightning Source LLC
Chambersburg PA
CBHW081719220526
45468CB00008B/1904